Trials of a Forensic Psychologist

Trials of a Forensic Psychologist

A CASEBOOK

Charles Patrick Ewing

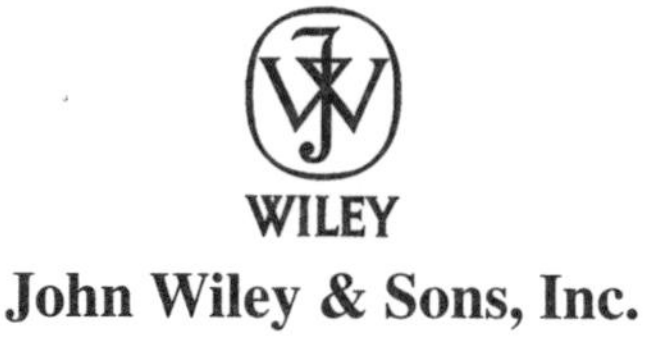

John Wiley & Sons, Inc.

This book is printed on acid-free paper.♾

Published by John Wiley & Sons, Inc., Hoboken, New Jersey.
Published simultaneously in Canada.

For general information on our other products and services please contact our Customer Care Department within the United States at (800) 762-2974, outside the United States at (317) 572-3993 or fax (317) 572-4002.

Wiley also publishes its books in a variety of electronic formats. Some content that appears in print may not be available in electronic books. For more information about Wiley products, visit our web site at www.wiley.com.

Library of Congress Cataloging-in-Publication Data:

Trials of a forensic psychologist: a casebook / by Charles Patrick Ewing.
p.; cm.
Includes bibliographical references and index.
ISBN 978-0-470-17072-4 (pbk.: alk. paper)
1. Forensic psychology—Case studies. I. Ewing, Charles Patrick, 1949–
[DNLM: 1. Crime—psychology—Case Reports. 2. Forensic Psychiatry—Case Reports. W 740 T819 2008]
RA1148.T75 2008
614′.15—dc22

2008008351

Printed in the United States of America.

10 9 8 7 6 5 4 3 2 1

To Sharon, my best friend.

CONTENTS

PREFACE

Twenty-five years ago, when I was a student at Harvard Law School, I worked for a semester at the office of a district attorney on Boston's north shore, prosecuting minor criminal and traffic cases under a state rule that allowed third-year law students to do so if supervised by experienced attorneys. One morning before heading to court to assist one of the prosecutors supervising my fieldwork, I was pulled aside by a secretary who asked if I minded answering a question. The question, delivered in a whisper, was: "I know this may sound stupid. But I've heard that you are a forensic psychologist. What does psychology have to do with dead bodies?"

The question was far from stupid, especially in the era before *CSI: Crime Scene Investigation* and today's public fascination with everything forensic. Suppressing a smile, I explained that the term *forensic* (though often associated with corpses, as in "forensic pathology") essentially means legal, and that forensic psychologists specialize in evaluating people involved in legal proceedings and sometimes testifying on their behalf or against them.

At the time the secretary posed her query, I was working on a law degree that I thought would complement my doctorate in psychology and give me an edge when it came to working in the emerging field of forensic psychology. For several years prior to attending law school, I had been working as a psychologist in a hospital, clinic, and private practice and found testifying in court to be a lot more stimulating and challenging than my everyday clinical work with patients.

I date my career as a forensic psychologist to my first experience on the witness stand about 30 years ago. I had finished my internship, completed my doctorate, done a postdoctoral fellowship, and was less than a year into my first real professional position in a hospital in Rochester, New York. Specializing at that time in the treatment of children and adolescents, I had been asked to evaluate a three-year-old girl who allegedly had been neglected by her parents. The local department of social services requested the evaluation to boost their chances in a lawsuit aimed at terminating the parents' rights to custody.

Psychological testing revealed that the girl had the mental capacity of a child half her chronological age—that is, about 18 months. My examinations of the parents were thorough but not difficult. The child's father was a chronic schizophrenic with few if any life skills and no parenting ability. Her mother was a severely dependent personality who, while not nearly as ill as her husband, was no more capable of parenting this or any child. The reports, which neither parent denied, indicated that the child had been found numerous times wandering the streets of inner-city Rochester and often seen hanging out of a third-story window. The family's apartment was filthy and infested with vermin. The refrigerator and cupboards were almost always empty. And the child slept on a urine-soaked mattress.

To me, the case was a no-brainer. I felt sorry for these folks but believed that they should have their parental rights to this child terminated. I was puzzled that my testimony would be needed to make that happen, but I gladly agreed to show up in family court and give my opinion.

I was, I subsequently learned, what lawyers call a "virgin expert." This was my first time out, and the attorney who presented my testimony felt that I would be more effective because it would be clear that I did not make a substantial portion of my living testifying. After an hour or so of questioning on direct examination, I certainly agreed. Smugly self-satisfied and more than a little self-righteous, I basked in the glow of the judge's enthusiastic smiles and nods as my direct testimony appeared to bury any chance these parents might have of maintaining custody of their child.

But then it all came apart. I had seen plenty of lawyer movies and TV shows, having grown up on *Perry Mason* and *The Defenders,* so I vaguely knew about cross-examination—the part of testimony when the opposing lawyer gets to question you. But anyone could see that this was an open-and-shut case, so what could the parents' attorney, a public defender, possibly do to shake my testimony?

The answer, as I learned over the next three hours that day and several more the next was: quite a lot. The parents' attorney, Charles Steinberg, who would later become my friend and mentor, ripped me, my evaluation, and my opinion from one end to the other. By the time he finished his withering cross-examination, even I was almost convinced that (1) I was a totally incompetent psychologist who had no business in the courtroom; and (2) that with appropriate social services these parents not only could but should be allowed to keep custody of their three-year-old.

That experience could easily have been both the beginning and end of my career as a forensic psychologist. As I have witnessed firsthand on many occasions since then, most of my mental health colleagues will do almost anything to avoid testifying, and those who do testify rarely if ever do so more than once.

But to my surprise, at the end of my testimony, the judge asked me if I would be willing to take court-appointed cases and testify as the court's witness; the social services attorney wondered if he could send more cases my way for evaluation; and Mr. Steinberg shook my hand, told me I'd been a worthy adversary, and asked if I would evaluate a couple of his clients at the public defender's office.

Talk about going from rags to riches; one moment I was silently swearing that I would never testify again, and the next thing I knew I was negotiating referrals that would undoubtedly put me right back in the witness chair.

At the time, I thought that I had somehow earned the confidence of this judge and these attorneys. Months later, with many more forensic cases under my belt, I said as much to Charlie Steinberg, who had by then already taken me under his wing and begun my education in law and reality. Charlie was kind but blunt. I got the cases from the court, the social services department, and his office, he said casually, not because I was good but because I was willing. Stick with it for a few years, he said, and I might get to be good at it.

I took Charlie's advice and soon was spending more time in court than in my clinical office. So much time, indeed, that I decided to go to law school to enhance my growing career as a forensic psychologist.

That was over 28 years ago. Since then, I have worked as a forensic psychologist in thousands of cases in dozens of states from New Hampshire to Hawaii and have testified in more than 600 trials.

This book recounts 10 trials, each a highly controversial case in which I gave expert testimony. My purpose here is to share some of my three decades of professional experience with students, colleagues, and other interested readers and to provide an inside, close-up look at what I have chosen to call the *Trials of a Forensic Psychologist*—a glimpse at the work of forensic psychologists, how their expertise is used (and sometimes abused) by the legal system, and the contributions they make to the system's ultimate goal of doing justice.

As will soon become apparent, the primary focus of this book is expert mental health testimony: the in-court examination and cross-examination of forensic psychologists by trial lawyers. It is the kind of book I wish I had available to me 30-some years ago before I first took the witness stand as an expert. It is the kind of book I would have appreciated years or even decades later. It is the kind of book I hope will be useful not only to students of psychology and law and aspiring and novice forensic psychologists and trial lawyers, but also to veteran practitioners in these fields who, like me, enjoy learning from the experiences (good and bad) of professional peers.

Author's Note

Forensic psychology—the application of psychological principles to legal issues—is both a private and public endeavor. Although there are some exceptions, forensic psychologists generally conduct evaluations of litigants behind closed doors and report their findings confidentially to attorneys. The attorneys, in collaboration with their clients, then decide whether and how to use these findings. Often, perhaps in the majority of cases, forensic psychological findings never go beyond this stage because they are not helpful to the legal position of the attorney and client who requested them. Examples include the criminal defendant who is evaluated and found to be sane, the personal injury litigant who is found not to have suffered significant psychological injury, and the civilly committed patient who is found to be in need of further inpatient care and treatment—to mention just a few.

Nevertheless, there are forensic psychological cases in which the findings of the psychologist become a matter of public record. These cases can provide rich teaching examples of the work of forensic psychologists—a chance to see how and why forensic psychologists reach the conclusions they do and how those conclusions are presented and challenged in court.

I have been a forensic psychologist for more than three decades, have conducted several thousand forensic evaluations, have testified in more than 600 trials, and have trained thousands of students, psychologists, lawyers, and judges in the practice of forensic psychology. Although my experience has certainly benefited me and the work I do—and I fervently hope that it has been beneficial to the cause of justice—it has often been difficult to translate that experience into something useful to students, colleagues, and others because so much of it has been part of the private or confidential realm of my work. Unless my work in a case has made it into the public realm, I have had to maintain confidentiality, and if I talked or wrote about a case at all, I could do so only on a limited, disguised basis. As a result, nearly all my vast professional experience has had little pedagogical use.

For many years, I have wanted to write a book such as this one—a volume in which I could go beyond brief and disguised anecdotes and offer a much richer, more interesting, and more pedagogically useful view of the work of a highly experienced forensic psychologist. My major concern—and the major obstacle to writing such a book—has always been confidentiality. Though often and necessarily sacrificed by our society's open legal process, confidentiality has been a cornerstone of forensic psychology. Thus, I could not, in either professional or personal conscience, write openly about most of the cases in which I have been involved.

My initial thought was to heavily disguise—and thus, to an extent, fictionalize—some of my cases in an effort to use those I thought would make the best teaching vehicles and still maintain the privacy and confidentiality of the individual litigants that I had evaluated. I quickly realized, however, that I would either sacrifice many of the very details that made those cases so fascinating and so ripe for teaching or run the risk that (because of their notoriety) their subjects would be immediately recognizable to at least some readers.

The alternative was to identify cases in which I have been involved that have become public as a result of testimony in open court and, in some instances, extensive media coverage. After many months of thought, discussion with colleagues, review of 30-plus years of case files, and reading of transcripts and media accounts of many of the cases in those files, I located 10 suitable cases in which there were sufficient public records of my work to enable me to write about them without disguising, fictionalizing, or distorting names, facts, conclusions, or any other aspect of the case.

In addition to this selection process, I should note several other important aspects of the writing of this book. First, the book is written in the first person, obviously by a participant-observer. While participant-observation is a time-honored research method, this work is not formal empirical research and is not intended to be read as such. Although my professional experience informs all my teaching, writing, and research, I was involved in these cases as a practicing professional, not as a researcher. While I have tried to be dispassionate and objective in my accounts of these cases, I would be the first to acknowledge that my professional involvement should caution any reader to question, not the accuracy of these accounts, but the reasons certain aspects of the cases are included or even highlighted, whereas others are limited or even omitted.

In advance, I offer a couple of explanations. To begin with, it is impossible to detail or even touch on every aspect of every case; readers who want more information about these cases would do well to read the transcripts and other public materials (books, news accounts, etc.) on which I have relied and have noted in the reference notes for each case. Also, I have scrupulously avoided mentioning information or aspects of these cases not available in the public record. Thus, although I have tried to give the reader a full and fair account of each case, I readily acknowledge that I know more about all these cases than I could write, even if I had an unlimited page budget. Moreover, like any author, I have tried to make my accounts not only accurate but interesting, critical, and thought-provoking. Naturally that means exercising a fair amount of editorial discretion.

Second, I make no claim that the cases included here are necessarily representative of the work of forensic psychologists in general; indeed, they are not fully representative of my own work as a forensic psychologist. All are criminal in nature. Forensic psychology is used in nearly every aspect of the legal system and is clearly not limited to criminal law issues. Again, the selection criteria previously noted were key factors; the nature and amount of public information in criminal prosecutions is generally much greater than that in other cases; indeed, in some areas of civil, family, and juvenile laws, even court records are unavailable.

Third, as will also become apparent to the reader, much of the public documentation used in writing this book came in the form of trial transcripts. Trial transcripts are verbatim records of in-court proceedings, made by highly skilled and certified court reporters. While they are usually accurate, they occasionally include typographical errors. Also, transcripts are written accounts of the spoken word, so they often read somewhat awkwardly. As much as possible, I have quoted directly from trial transcripts rather than trying to characterize what was said. This approach means that many of the chapters in this volume are replete with extensive direct quotations from trial transcripts. With a few exceptions that were made for purposes of clarity (and are appropriately marked with brackets or ellipses), I have quoted the transcript as written. As a result, a number of these quotes (including some of my own) do not include the best or, in some instances, even proper grammar and punctuation. I trust that the reader will understand the difficulty of being fully articulate when testifying or asking questions of a witness in the heat of courtroom battle.

Despite these caveats, I hope that readers will find these case studies informative, educational, and compelling.

ACKNOWLEDGMENTS

It is impossible to properly thank all the people who have contributed to this book. First and foremost are the thousands of people who have made my career as a forensic psychologist possible. While only a handful of their stories have made it into this volume, each has taught me something and enriched my career and, I like to think, has deepened not only my understanding of forensic psychology but also my humanity.

It is also impossible to individually thank the countless lawyers from whom I have learned the finer points of my profession as they have examined and cross-examined me on the witness stand. Those mentioned by name in this book—Charles Steinberg, Joel Daniels, John Nuchereno, William Sullivan, Robert French, Paul Carbonaro, John Speranza, Charles Siragusa, Robert Simpson, Robert Miller, Raymond Urbanski, Felix Lapine, Robin Shellow, George Quinlan, Michael Vavonese, Paul Cleary, and the late George Dentes have all—intentionally or otherwise—taught me valuable lessons about how to be a more effective expert witness. Likewise, many of my fellow experts, including those mentioned in this book—Barbara Miller, Thomas Lazzaro, Richard Ciccone, Dewey Cornell, and the late Russell Barton—have all taught me similarly valuable lessons.

All these people and countless others helped prepare me to write this book and I sincerely thank them all.

When it came to actually writing the book, fewer people were of direct assistance, but in many ways their help was even more valuable. Among the standouts who deserve my deepest gratitude are:

- Patricia Rossi, Executive Editor for Psychology at John Wiley & Sons, Inc. "Tisha" saw the merit to this book and helped the publisher see it as well.
- Andrea Ott, a JD-PhD student in law and philosophy. Andrea was as dedicated a research assistant as any author could ever ask for. Andrea and her successor, Laura Scheestel, another law student, spared no effort in tracking down and obtaining transcripts and other public records of the cases about which I have written.
- Susan Martin, my administrative assistant and manager and protector of my working life at the University at Buffalo. Sue oversaw the work of Andrea, Laura, and other students who contributed many hours of their time to the research needed to make this book possible.
- My colleagues, Drs. Alan Goldstein, Robert Fein, Gerald Koocher, Randy Otto, David Shapiro, Paul Lipsett, and Robert Meyer. Each of these leading forensic psychologists generously took time out of their busy schedules as professors and practitioners to field my questions and offer me advice and counsel in the preparation of this book.
- My wife and partner in all things, Dr. Sharon Harris-Ewing. Sharon has lived through it all with me, and I could not have done any of it without her.

Trials of a Forensic Psychologist

CHAPTER 1

Waiver of Miranda *Rights and Voluntary versus Coerced Confession*

1

You don't have to be a psychologist to know that a stressful life prematurely ages you and takes a terrible toll on your physical and mental health. That was certainly true for Waneta Hoyt.

When I first met her, in 1994, Waneta was 47 years old, but she could easily have passed for 65. Pale, frail, and gaunt, she moved slowly and deliberately, as if in constant pain or perhaps in fear of a crippling fall. Much of Waneta's hair had fallen out, and what little was left was thin, wispy, and of indeterminate color. Thick, oversized eyeglasses obscured much of her face and gave her a perpetually bewildered look. Always feeling either too warm or too cold, she dressed oddly, which added to the illusion of senior citizenship.

Waneta attributed her constant discomfort with the temperature to a circulatory disorder, but she also suffered from high blood pressure, arthritis, osteoporosis, borderline diabetes, angina, allergies, chronic depression, swelling in her feet, and numbness in her hands. She could not climb a flight of stairs and found it hard to walk more than a couple of hundred yards without becoming short of breath or falling. As a result, she was virtually housebound, leaving home alone only to do necessary errands such as picking up the mail or driving her 17-year-old son Jay to school.

Physically and psychologically, Waneta was almost completely dependent on her husband, Tim. She, Tim, and Jay lived in a small rented house near Owego in rural upstate New York and barely got by financially on Tim's meager earnings as a part-time Pinkerton's security guard at nearby Cornell University. The couple had a bank balance of five dollars, had twice filed for bankruptcy, and were one missed paycheck away from homelessness.

One of Waneta's sisters was dying from a brain tumor, while another battled cancer. Both were partially paralyzed and confined to wheelchairs. Five years earlier, Waneta's mother had been killed in a car accident. In 1973, Waneta had been raped by a neighbor. That same year, her mobile home burned, and she and Tim lost everything but the clothes on their backs. In 1964, the year she and Tim married, her father-in-law hanged himself.

But those traumas paled by comparison to the ones that ultimately led Waneta to my office. Between 1965 and 1971, Waneta gave birth to five children, Eric, Julie, James, Molly, and Noah, each of whom died at ages ranging from 48 days to 28 months, victims of what medical authorities said was sudden infant death syndrome (SIDS).

For the next two decades and more, Waneta quietly lived with her grief and gradually became a recluse. Family, friends, and neighbors alike regarded her as the victim of a tragedy beyond comprehension, a pathetic soul afflicted with a rare but fatal and probably genetically transmitted disease that killed any child to whom she gave birth. That perception was reinforced when, some years after the death of their fifth child, Waneta and Tim adopted a baby boy. Jay, their adopted son, was healthy throughout infancy and childhood and had grown into adolescence and the verge of adulthood with no problems.

In all likelihood, the story of Waneta Hoyt and her five dead babies would have remained nothing more than a personal calamity had it not been for the scientific curiosity of a young physician who treated Molly and Noah, the fourth- and fifth-born Hoyt children, prior to their deaths.

At the time, Dr. Alfred Steinschneider was a research pediatrician investigating the relationship of apnea (sporadic involuntary pauses in breathing) to SIDS at the Upstate Medical Center in Syracuse, 70 miles from the Hoyts' home. Steinschneider noted Molly and Noah's extraordinary histories: Each had experienced periods of apnea, died suddenly and inexplicably from what was characterized as SIDS, and had four siblings with similar histories, including sudden and unexplained death in infancy or very early childhood.

Prior to their early deaths, both Molly and Noah had been hospitalized, treated, studied by Steinschneider, and found to present multiple instances of prolonged apnea. Relying on data from their cases, as well as from three other unrelated infants, in 1972, Steinschneider published a groundbreaking research report in the prestigious medical journal *Pediatrics*. In "Prolonged Apnea and the Sudden Infant Death Syndrome," he presented data supporting his hypothesis that SIDS was caused by prolonged apnea and had a strong familial, genetic basis.[1] The short lives and sudden deaths of Molly and Noah Hoyt, identified only as M.H. and N.H., were described in detail in the article, which also mentioned the apparent SIDS deaths of their three siblings.

While Waneta and Tim Hoyt watched their lives spiral into poverty and despair, Dr. Steinschneider went on to become perhaps the world's leading authority on SIDS. His seminal article spawned a federally funded research empire that led to the widespread use of in-home apnea monitors with infants thought to be at risk for SIDS. These devices, which Steinschneider had first home-tested with Molly and Noah, kept constant track of infant breathing and alerted parents to any evidence of apnea.

But Steinschneider's theory was not without its critics. Indeed, publication of his article in *Pediatrics* was followed quickly by a harshly critical letter to the editor of the esteemed journal in which Dr. John Hick noted that prolonged apnea did not adequately explain the infants' symptoms, much less their deaths. More significantly, Hick took Steinschneider to task for failing to consider the possibility that the children's deaths were the result of foul play:

> Despite the circumstantial evidence suggesting a critical role for the mother in the death of her children Steinschneider offers no information about the woman. . . . The potential for child abuse inherent in the family history . . . could have been more adequately controlled in this study, had Steinschneider only chosen a foster home as his laboratory for the investigation of the youngest sibling. Perhaps the outcome would have been different?[2]

As if the point were not made sufficiently by Hick's scathing letter, *Pediatrics* received and published a second letter from Dr. Vincent DiMaio, a medical examiner and author of a well-known textbook on forensic pathology. DiMaio wrote that, based on his reading of the Steinschneider article, the five "H" children's deaths were "in all medical probability homicides by smothering."[3] DiMaio added that in his experience, "The perpetrator is virtually always the mother and she will continue this killing unless stopped or until she runs out of children."[4] Later, in his text, *Forensic Pathology,* DiMaio was even more blunt and accusatory:

> The association of SIDS with apneic episodes as an entity was brought to prominence in an article by Steinschneider. A review of this paper indicates that his two reported cases of sudden infant death associated with prolonged apnea were siblings and probably victims of homicides, as were prior siblings.[5]

Steinschneider's theory of SIDS was hotly debated in the years following publication of his article in *Pediatrics*. That debate, however, was largely academic, if not esoteric, and confined to a relatively small group of interested medical professionals. And so it remained until 1986, when an obscure Texas medical examiner was called to consult on a possible case of infanticide in Syracuse, the city in which Steinschneider had treated and studied the Hoyt children and from whose medical center he published "Prolonged Apnea and the Sudden Infant Death Syndrome." The Texas pathologist, long aware of the article and the controversy it had generated in the medical community, warned a Syracuse prosecutor, William Fitzpatrick, that he might have a serial killer on the loose in his community. Dr. Linda Norton of Dallas told Fitzpatrick:

> Steinschneider writes this idiotic paper . . . and he says the two babies that he studied had spells of prolonged apnea before they died. And so therefore the implication is that apnea causes SIDS and SIDS is familial. . . . It's always been clear to me that these babies were smothered, probably by their mother, because she seems to be the one reporting the incidents. . . . Steinschneider [has] built an entire theory of Sudden Infant Death Syndrome on homicides. And that woman's right here in Syracuse.[6]

In 1992, 20 years after publication of the *Pediatrics* article and six years after listening to Norton's disdain for Steinschneider and his research, Fitzpatrick decided to look into the case. After reading Steinschneider's article, Fitzpatrick felt that Norton might have been right. A few phone calls and a little digging revealed the surnames of the "H" children, and confidential hospital records led to their parents: Waneta and Tim Hoyt.

If Fitzpatrick could make a case against Waneta after all these years, it would be the achievement of a lifetime and bring him more fame than a little-known small town district attorney (DA) could have ever hoped to attain. To Fitzpatrick's chagrin, however, further investigation revealed that the Hoyt children had died, not in Onondaga County, where he had jurisdiction, but two counties away in Tioga County where the DA was a man named Robert Simpson.

Fitzpatrick contacted Simpson and outlined his theory of the case: five babies dead, all wrongly diagnosed as having succumbed to SIDS; and a mother who had gotten away with murder, still living in Simpson's county.

Over a year later, Fitzpatrick had received no reply from Simpson, who was understandably reluctant to spend the extremely scarce resources of his small, impoverished county to look into the long-stale case. By the summer of 1993, Fitzpatrick was fuming. "I haven't heard anything, goddamn it," he complained. "I can't believe I handed this guy the case of his life and I haven't heard anything."[7] Finally, 15 months after his first contact with Simpson, Fitzpatrick wrote to the small-county DA, threatening to assert jurisdiction over the case on the legally dubious grounds that Waneta had taken two of her children to the Syracuse hospital prior to their deaths.

Simpson got the message and directed the New York State Police to begin investigating the Hoyt saga. Prosecutors and investigators talked to several pathologists who told them essentially that the deaths of the Hoyt babies virtually had to have been homicides, even though none was ever so classified.

Among those consulted was Dr. Michael Baden, who would later become famous for his role in the defense of alleged murderer O.J. Simpson. Baden was the former New York City medical examiner and significantly—at the time of the Hoyt investigation—co-director of the crime lab of the New York State Police, the agency investigating the case. After reviewing only the decades-old paper trail in the case, Baden offered his assessment:

> [T]he causes of death are wrong. That's number one. I see no evidence of natural disease. Number two is the pattern of deaths. The age of the two-and-a-half-year-old, who could not be a SIDS death, and the circumstances of the individual cases indicate they were suffocated.[8]

Bolstered by the pathologist's seeming certainty that the Hoyt children could not have died by means other than homicide, even though their deaths had all been medically certified at the time as the result of natural causes, the investigative team left no stone unturned in their efforts to develop a profile of Waneta and Tim Hoyt, a dossier they hoped would assure that, when questioned, Waneta would confess to having killed her five children.

New York State Police officers obtained Waneta's medical and mental health records, the medical records of Tim, and even those of the couple's teenage son Jay. They scoured the Hoyts' employment records, credit reports, driving records, and utility bills. The investigators even went so far as to secure a "mail cover" that allowed them to examine the outside of the Hoyts' incoming and outgoing mail and a telephone tap that recorded any numbers the Hoyts called.

The investigators also consulted with a forensic psychologist and sought his advice on how best to get Waneta to confess when they ultimately confronted her with the evidence against her. The psychologist, who worked for the state department of mental health, eagerly joined the team and lent his expertise, suggesting, among other things, that the investigators take pains to make Waneta feel emotionally safe even while she was at obvious legal peril.

After numerous calls, meetings, and strategy sessions, the long-awaited confrontation was set. On March 23, 1994, the State Police would finally go head-to-head with the woman they were certain was a serial child murderer. They knew the stakes were high, that this would be their one shot at obtaining a confession from Waneta, and that without such a confession, all their work would likely go for naught. As two reporters who interviewed the lead officer, Robert Courtright, later explained, "Courtright felt the window of opportunity would be small, especially if Mrs. Hoyt claimed innocence and got herself a lawyer who would immediately tell her to keep her mouth shut and circle the wagons. That would be some infernal public spectacle, Courtright thought. He could just imagine the headlines . . . Newark Valley Mom Claims Witch Hunt."[9]

Despite Courtright's worries, the interrogation plan worked like a charm. Waneta was approached first by "Bubba" Bleck, a local police officer she had known, liked, and trusted for years. Bleck located Waneta near the post office early in the morning and introduced her to Susan Mulvey, a State Police officer who had been designated to do most of the interrogation.

Mulvey, a 15-year veteran of the state force and the only woman in her troop's 45-member investigative division, was strategically dressed for the occasion, wearing a plain blue suit and a locket bearing the photo of her own infant daughter. Bleck told Waneta that Mulvey was an "investigator," that she was helping a medical doctor in Minnesota with a study of SIDS, knew about Waneta's babies' deaths, and wanted to interview her. Mulvey told Waneta, "We'd like to talk to you about how your children died. You'd be the best person to talk to because you were there."[10] Then, adding a lie, Mulvey said, "The records aren't around."[11]

Finally, in a well-planned effort to secure Waneta's cooperation, Mulvey continued to prevaricate, telling the gullible murder suspect, "We heard about your children from a medical article written by Dr. Steinschneider from Syracuse. And we've talked to a doctor from Minnesota about it and looked at the medical records. But the information is a little sketchy to us, so we'd like to know a little bit more and you're the best person to talk to because you were there. I've been assigned to get as much information as possible about how your babies lived and died, and the reason I'm doing it and not the doctors is that this isn't their area of expertise. This is what I do every day, talk to people. That's why they asked me to talk to you. So maybe we can prevent this from happening to other children. Would you be willing to talk to us?"[12]

Waneta readily agreed. If it would "help anyone else," Waneta said, she would be glad to be interviewed.[13] As she would recall later—and entirely plausibly from her perspective—she believed that she was being invited to take part in a research project dealing with SIDS.

After a quick trip back to Waneta's home to pick up her son and take him to school, Bleck and Mulvey took Waneta in an unmarked car to the Owego State Police barracks, where she was to be interrogated. Unknown to Waneta, at the same time, other State Police officers were carrying out a prearranged plan to detain and question Tim Hoyt at his job at Cornell. Tim was assigned by Pinkerton's as a security guard at the university's art museum. The plan, which was executed that morning, was to remove Tim from the job site, thereby making him inaccessible if Waneta happened to call him. On the pretense that they were investigating stolen artwork, two officers took Tim to the State Police barracks in Ithaca, where they began questioning him about the deaths of his children.

Meanwhile, back at the Owego barracks, Waneta was placed in a small room with Bleck, Mulvey, and Courtright; quickly given her *Miranda* rights (told that she had the right to remain silent, that anything she said could be used against her in court, and that she had the right to have a lawyer present); and asked if she understood and agreed to talk. Then, in what appears to have been an effort to maintain the SIDS research charade, Officer Bleck falsely reassured Waneta that giving the warning was standard procedure whenever anyone was interviewed at the police barracks. As police officers are trained and well know, *Miranda* warnings need be given only to suspects who are in custody. Everybody in the room but Waneta knew that she was a suspect and that she was in custody. Only Waneta believed that what was about to happen had anything to do with research on SIDS.

Since the police failed to videotape or even make an audio record of the interrogation, what followed depends on whose version of the facts you accept. There is no dispute that, by late that afternoon, the police had their coveted confession, a handwritten statement signed by Waneta and a later question-and-answer session taken down and transcribed by a freelance court reporter. For good measure, and obvious self-serving reasons, Mulvey even got Waneta to add an addendum to her confession: "The people here have been kind in this matter."[14]

The question was not whether Waneta confessed, but why and whether her confession was truthful.

According to the police, Mulvey spent most of the morning encouraging Waneta to tell her story of the lives and deaths of her children, much the same way as a genuine SIDS researcher might have gone about the task. But then, after a short break, Mulvey confronted Waneta, telling her, "The medical evidence shows that you did something to cause the children to die."[15] That statement was false, of course, because at best the pathologists surmised that Waneta's babies had been suffocated. There was no medical evidence of that, much less any proof that, if they had been killed, Waneta was the culprit.

According to the police account, Waneta balked briefly, referring Mulvey to Dr. Steinschneider, but then quickly confessed to killing all five of her children. Tim Hoyt was brought to the Owego barracks and confronted with Waneta's confession, which she eventually signed with him as a witness. Waneta was then questioned under oath by

Courtright in front of the court reporter and repeated much of her earlier confession.

Waneta was arrested and jailed that afternoon, but the ink on the confession was barely dry before she renounced it. She had a different account of how the incriminating statement came about. She recalled Bleck reading her *Miranda* rights from a card she was unable to read on her own because she was without her reading glasses. She heard the words he recited but didn't listen because she thought she was there for a research interview and because Bleck assured her that this was simply a formality. She was eager to cooperate and said she understood what was read aloud to her even though she did not.

Waneta recalled the first part of the interrogation much as the police described it. Hoping to be helpful, she gave the police a detailed account of the lives and deaths of her children. But, after the break, Mulvey took her by the hands and told her that the police had concrete proof that she had suffocated her babies. Mulvey repeatedly told her that she killed her children. Waneta denied the accusations, but Mulvey wouldn't take "no" for an answer. Instead, Mulvey began stroking Waneta's arms. Bleck put his arm around Waneta's shoulders while Mulvey disingenuously told her that she was there to help her. Mulvey then suggested various scenarios for each of the deaths, such as smothering the children with pillows, that fit with the pathologists' speculations.

According to Waneta, she kept saying "no"—denying that she had killed her children—until Mulvey wore her down: "She said I must have done it because they have this concrete medical proof, and I said, no, I didn't. I didn't. And they just kept at me for I don't know how long. And finally I says, 'Yeah, I guess I did. If you say I did.'"[16]

What do you do when you are an attorney representing a client who has confessed to multiple homicides but recants her confession and tells you that she was fed the confession by her interrogators and pushed into confessing? Waneta's two public defenders, Robert Miller and Raymond Urbanski, were experienced and knowledgeable criminal defense attorneys. They knew enough not to trust everything a client told them but also never to trust everything the police claimed. They knew that since the police could produce no direct proof that Waneta killed her children, her confession would be the crucial piece of evidence against her. They knew that there was a large body of psychological literature documenting false confessions and the tactics used by the police to obtain them. And, perhaps most significantly, they knew that despite their years of experience and expertise, they were in over their heads with regard to the confession. They needed an expert, a psychologist who could evaluate the confession, examine and test Waneta, and help answer the critical legal questions: Did Waneta make a knowing and intelligent waiver of her *Miranda* rights, and was her confession voluntary?

It took Miller and Urbanski just a few calls to come up with my name. At the time, there were no other board-certified forensic psychologists in upstate New York and perhaps only one other in the entire state. Indeed, there were then only about 150 of us in the nation, and I was among the very few who had often dealt with the issues confronting them. Moreover, at the time, I was working on a major project researching homicides within families and had testified in many such cases. Unknown to Miller and Urbanski, I also had more than a passing acquaintance with SIDS, having served as president and a member of the board of directors of a regional SIDS foundation many years earlier.

On June 27, 1994, just three months after her arrest, Waneta Hoyt showed up at my office, approximately 150 miles from her home. That was the first of the nine times I would interview her over a period of eight months prior to her trial. Before the evaluation was complete, I would also conduct objective psychological testing with Waneta.

By the time I first met Waneta, I had reviewed hundreds of pages of documents, including the handwritten confession and the transcript of Waneta's Q&A with Officer Courtright. The first thing I noticed when looking over the confession was that, except for the addendum requested by Mulvey about how well Waneta had been treated by the police, the document was not in Waneta's handwriting. The confession was neatly penned in precise, businesslike, completely legible printing that could not possibly be mistaken for Waneta's shaky scrawl. It was also entirely grammatically correct, properly punctuated, and clearly written in what I immediately recognized as *cop-speak,* not the language of a high school dropout who'd had only one real job in her entire life. The first line read as follows: "I caused the death of all my five (5) children."[17] I am no expert in handwriting, but comparing the writing in the statement to that of Waneta and Mulvey, it seemed evident to me that the statement Waneta had signed was written by Mulvey, who also signed it as a witness.

There was also something immediately troubling about the transcript of Courtright's session with Waneta. A portion of the Q&A dealing with the death of Eric, Waneta's firstborn child, read as follows:

Q: What happened?

A: I took a pillow and suffocated him, I guess . . .

Q: When you put the pillow over Eric's face, did that cause his death?

A: I guess so, yes.[18]

Waneta had been interrogated for hours on end, signed a written detailed confession, and now was "guessing" about what she had done to her children?

Meeting, interviewing, testing, and getting to know Waneta made me even more skeptical of the state's position that she knowingly and intelligently waived her *Miranda* rights and that she voluntarily confessed to killing five infants. My assessment of Waneta, which involved 21 hours of face-to-face interviewing and testing, led me to conclude that she suffered from long-standing, recurring episodes of serious depression as well as severe dependent and avoidant personality disorders.

The symptoms of these personality disorders, as described in the American Psychiatric Association's *Diagnostic and Statistical Manual of Mental Disorders*, painted an almost perfect picture of Waneta Hoyt:

> The essential feature of Dependent Personality Disorder is a pervasive and excessive need to be taken care of that leads to submissive and clinging behavior and fears of separation. . . .
>
> Individuals with Dependent Personality Disorder have great difficulty making everyday decisions . . . without an excessive amount of advice

> and reassurance from others. These individuals tend to be passive and to allow other people (often a single other person) to take the initiative and assume responsibility for most major areas of their lives. . . . Because they fear losing support or approval, individuals with Dependent Personality Disorder often have difficulty expressing disagreement with other people. . . . These individuals feel so unable to function alone that they will agree with things that they feel are wrong rather than risk losing the help of those to whom they look for guidance. . . .
>
> Individuals with Dependent Personality Disorder may go to excessive lengths to obtain nurturance and support from others, even to the point of volunteering for unpleasant tasks if such behavior will bring the care they need. . . . They are willing to submit to what others want, even if the demands are unreasonable. . . .
>
> The essential feature of Avoidant Personality Disorder is a pervasive pattern of social inhibition, feelings of inadequacy, and hypersensitivity to negative evaluation that begins by early adulthood and is present in a variety of contexts.
>
> Individuals with Avoidant Personality Disorder avoid work or school activities that involve significant interpersonal contact because of fears of criticism, disapproval, or rejection. . . .
>
> Individuals with Avoidant Personality Disorder are inhibited in new interpersonal situations because they feel inadequate and have low self-esteem. Doubts concerning social competence and personal appeal become especially manifest in settings involving interactions with strangers. These individuals believe themselves to be socially inept, personally unappealing, and inferior to others.[19]

This personality profile was reinforced by the objective psychological testing, which revealed that Waneta felt unhappy, weak, and fatigued much of the time; was docile, passive, and overly dependent; felt inadequate, insecure, and helpless; lacked interest and involvement in life; looked to others for nurturance and support; wanted to be seen in a positive light by others; and was easily hurt even by mild criticism.

Putting Waneta's personality and psychopathology together with the circumstances of her interrogation and confession, I concluded that, whatever happened to her children, she did not voluntarily confess to killing them.

As I would learn much later, during the course of my evaluation of Waneta, her attorneys sought another opinion from a prominent British psychologist, Dr. Gisli Gudjonsson, who had written an important book called *The Psychology of Interrogations, Confessions, and Testimony.* At the request of the public defenders, Gudjonsson had flown to upstate New York and conducted his own brief evaluation of Waneta and her confession. When he had completed his work with Waneta, Gudjonsson visited my office with one of Waneta's attorneys, and we had what I thought was a confidential meeting. Gudjonsson and I discussed the case at some length and, in order not to bias our conclusions, neither of us revealed our findings to the other. Since the contents of this meeting were never revealed by me or made part of the public record through testimony or reports revealed in court, I am not at liberty to say what took place.

However, in a later popular exposé, two newspaper reporters purported to reveal the contents of that meeting. According to them, after evaluating Waneta, Gudjonsson told Miller and Urbanski "I'm afraid I'm not going to be able to help you. . . . She's manipulating everybody, and if you had me testify, I'd have to say those statements to the police are perfectly reliable."[20] According to these reporters, Waneta's attorneys were worried that if I found out that Gudjonsson disagreed with me, I might change my opinion. Thus, according to their account, the attorneys convinced Gudjonsson to meet with me "and perhaps encourage [me] to keep thinking Waneta was innocent."[21] The reporters cited Waneta's lawyers as their source and quoted both men by name.

I was not thinking in terms of innocence or guilt when I met with Gudjonsson. My job was only to determine whether Waneta's confession was voluntarily given. Later, when the reporters published their account, I e-mailed Gudjonsson and asked if the accounts of his opinion and his purported effort to manipulate me were accurate. Gudjonsson responded quickly: "Thank you for your e-mail. The comments attributed to me are false. . . . I did not make any attempt to manipulate you in any way at our meeting, nor did I discuss doing so with anybody. For anybody to do so would be totally unethical. . . . My advice to [her attorney] was to focus on the ways in which Mrs. Hoyt had been manipulated by the police and her legal rights apparently violated."[22]

Though I reported my findings to Waneta's attorneys well in advance of the trial, I later learned that they waited until the last minute to spring my report and anticipated testimony on Robert Simpson, the district attorney prosecuting Waneta. Given the state of New York law at that time, this was neither improper nor bad strategy. The law has since changed, but then required pretrial notice of the defense's intent to present expert psychological testimony only where the defendant was relying on a psychological defense such as insanity or extreme emotional disturbance. Here, of course, my testimony would not support any such defense but rather lend ammunition to an attack on the admissibility of Waneta's confession.

When, late in the trial, Simpson learned about my involvement and expected testimony, he was outraged. "I look like the village idiot," he told the judge, complaining that he had been sandbagged by the late notice, would not have time to prepare to cross-examine me effectively, and would not be able to have Waneta examined by an expert of his choosing.[23] Despite Simpson's reasoned arguments, the judge ruled properly that I would be allowed to testify because my testimony would go not to her state of mind at the time of the alleged crimes but rather at the time of the confession. In fairness to Simpson, the judge adjourned court for a day, Friday, thus allowing the prosecutor a long weekend to find an expert of his own and find someone to help him prepare to cross-examine me.

Simpson called the state-employed forensic psychologist who earlier assisted in developing the police strategy for Waneta's interrogation. The psychologist not only directed the prosecutor to a psychiatrist who (amazingly, in my experience) would do the evaluation on a moment's notice, but also tutored the DA on how to cross-examine me.

Fresh from a hastily arranged, two-hour interview with the prosecution's newly found expert, Waneta took the stand in her own defense and described her tragic life, including the deaths of her children, the interrogation, and her arrest. She denied killing her children. Apparently this is exactly what Waneta wanted—the chance to tell her side of the story—because, according to later journalistic accounts of the case, she could probably have pleaded guilty to lesser charges and been sentenced to a short period of incarceration or perhaps even probation; but she refused to consider any plea bargain whatsoever.

Waneta was followed to the witness stand by her husband and son, neither of whom added much substance to the case. Then it was time for my testimony. By then, the jury had already heard from expert witnesses for both sides, debating the question of how the Hoyt children died. Even if the prosecution won that round, managing to show that the children's deaths were homicides, it needed Waneta's confession to pin the alleged killings on her. At the end of the trial, the jury would be instructed by the judge that if they determined that Waneta had not voluntarily confessed, they would have no choice but to completely ignore her confession. In that case, given the state of the evidence, they would also have little choice but to acquit Waneta.

Thus, not surprisingly, Waneta and her attorneys had a lot riding on my testimony. I had conducted a thorough (21-plus hour) evaluation of the defendant and had plenty of experience on the witness stand, having previously testified in over 400 trials for both the prosecution and the defense. I felt confident about my role in the trial, but I did not share the optimism of Waneta and her lawyers. I knew from experience that jurors often give little weight to the testimony of psychological experts, especially those called by the defense. My experience had taught me that in criminal trials jurors often regard prosecution witnesses as objective professionals doing a public service, while they see defense experts as hired guns who would say anything for the right amount of money.

To help overcome that bias, Ray Urbanski began his questioning with my credentials (Cornell PhD, Yale postdoctoral fellow, Harvard law degree, tenured full professor, journal editor, expert witness for both sides, etc.). The idea was to undercut the unfortunate bias that exists against experts called by the defense. I agreed that as a matter of standard practice we had to do it, but worried (as I always do) that it might backfire. The jurors were ordinary small-town folks who might look at me as some kind of highly paid, self-important, big city hotshot brought in to tell them what to do. What I would like them to have known, but couldn't tell them, was that I wasn't born with an Ivy League pedigree but had entered this world just 20 miles down the road, where I was raised by a single mother who, though she worked long and hard, was as poor as the Hoyts and usually finished the week with less than a quarter to her name.

Once Urbanski established my credentials and qualified me to testify as an expert, I slowly went through all that I had learned about the case from Waneta and the records I had reviewed. Not surprisingly, Simpson objected repeatedly, trying in vain to get the judge to cut me off because much of what I was saying the jury was hearing for the first time. The judge said he was giving me wide latitude and reminded Simpson that he could cross-examine me and try to rebut my testimony with that of his own expert.

Ultimately, Urbanski asked me how my findings regarding Waneta's personality disorders related to the techniques employed by the police in trying to get her to confess. I explained, "She was particularly vulnerable to the use of a man she thought was her friend, Officer Bleck, to induce her cooperation to begin with. She was vulnerable to the misrepresentation to her about the true nature of the interview, that this was a SIDS interview rather than a police interrogation, that giving this interview would somehow be helpful to research on SIDS. She was vulnerable to the lying to her about the purpose of the *Miranda* warning, having been told that this was routine in these kinds of situations. I believe she was especially vulnerable to the use of a female investigator, accompanied by two male authority figures. I also believe that she was extremely vulnerable to the touching and the rubbing of her body and that this lowered her resistance and induced greater cooperation. I also think that she was extremely vulnerable to the repeated verbal demands, the insistence that she actually did kill her children when she said she didn't. She was also vulnerable to her own feelings of guilt about not having done more over the years somehow to have helped her children live. And finally I think she was perhaps most vulnerable of all to the fact that she was isolated from her husband, the person upon whom she was totally dependent."[24]

Finally, in response to the defense lawyer's last question, I told the jury, "It is my conclusion that her statement to the police on that day was not made knowingly, and it was not made voluntarily."[25]

Simpson, who had been seething throughout my direct testimony, now seemed beside himself with anger and indignation. He seemed to take my testimony as some kind of personal affront. He accused me of tailoring my testimony to fit the defense because I was being paid by the Public Defender's Office, apparently forgetting that his own expert witness was being paid even more by the DA's Office. He made much of the fact that I had not seen a handful of 20-year-old psychiatric records that were not available to me. He implied that Waneta had fabricated her responses to the psychological testing, which he apparently did not realize had built-in measures of validity, testing that was not even undertaken by his own expert. Finally, in a state close to rage, he demanded that I tell the jury what the police had done wrong in this case.

Simpson was angry but not stupid. When I started to answer his question, he caught himself and objected. When Urbanski complained that Simpson was, in essence, objecting to his own question, the judge agreed and directed me to finish.

The trial's last witness was Dr. David Barry, the psychiatrist who had examined Waneta for the DA just a week before. I knew of Barry by reputation. He was an experienced and competent practitioner. But, with all due respect for his competence, I had to wonder what he could really say in a complex case like this based on a one-time, two-hour, totally subjective, and hastily arranged interview for which he had made himself available with virtually no advance notice.

When I thought about how the prosecutor had gotten Barry's name, the more cynical part of me recalled what I often tell my students about why prosecutors have to be extremely careful in selecting expert witnesses. Under our system of criminal justice, if the defense attorney hires an expert and that expert does not support the attorney's case, the attorney merely pays the expert and says goodbye. But if the prosecutor hires an expert who renders an opinion that favors the defendant, the prosecutor must turn that opinion over to the defense attorney, who, if he chooses, may then call that expert as his own witness and, of course, ask the expert who hired him in the first place.

Though Barry had done no psychological testing of Waneta's personality, he told the jury that she suffered no personality disorders. But on cross-examination, one of Waneta's attorneys presented the prosecution psychiatrist with a hypothetical question based on the circumstances of Waneta's confession. Given those circumstances, the defense attorney asked if it would be significant that the person interrogated by the police thought she was participating in a research interview. Like his direct testimony, Barry's answer was straightforward: "If that's the way it happened, I'd say there was some significance. Your hypothetical describes a situation in which Mrs. Hoyt was clearly anticipating quite a different course for the discussion than the one it eventually took."[26] As a reporter covering the trial wrote, "Barry had essentially agreed with Ewing: If police had told Waneta they wanted to talk to her for SIDS research, then she had been manipulated."[27]

In his closing argument, defense attorney Robert Miller hammered away at this point, noting the essential agreement of the two experts and arguing that Waneta's constitutional rights had been violated by the police. On the other hand, prosecutor Robert Simpson pinned his hopes on the medical evidence and appeared to throw in the towel on the confession issue. "Forget the confession," he told the jury. "There is something wrong here. You can take some of these things away, and you wouldn't be suspicious. If the children had these life-threatening problems in the hospital, we wouldn't be here today. If there were other people in the neighborhood who had seen these problems, we wouldn't be here today. If we had some sickness we could see for these children, if we had some hospital record that showed them as other than normal, healthy children, we wouldn't be here today. But the coincidences mount and mount in this case, so we don't have coincidences anymore."[28]

In the final analysis, the jury agreed with Simpson's assessment of the evidence. Over the course of two days of deliberations, several jurors expressed serious concern about the tactics and tricks the police used to get Waneta to confess. They spent half their deliberations considering whether the confession should be suppressed before concluding that it should not. In whatever manner it may have been obtained, the jury concluded that Waneta's confession was true. And that, coupled with the debatable medical testimony, was enough for them to convict her on all five counts of murder.

Act one of this morality play was over. Act two would be much shorter but not without its own high drama and surprise ending. Found guilty in April 1995, Waneta was not scheduled for sentencing until June 23. Meanwhile, she was remanded without bail to the Tioga County Jail, where she had little else to do but obsess over her fate. In early May, Waneta wrote a letter to the judge who had presided over her trial and was soon to sentence her. In the letter, Waneta complained that she had been "railroaded" and badly represented by her attorneys.[29] The judge did not respond but passed the correspondence to the attorneys. Several weeks later, Waneta wrote the judge again, complaining about her lawyers and begging not to be sent to prison. When the judge still did not respond, Waneta got his attention with another missive, this time informing him that she wanted to fire her lawyers. "I regret to say that these two gentlemen misrepresented me in my trial," she wrote just three weeks before she was to be sentenced.[30]

On the day Waneta was to be sentenced, the judge gave her the opportunity to explain herself. Although he could find no fault with the way she had been represented, the judge allowed Waneta to dismiss her attorneys. The judge warned her that by firing the public defenders, she was giving up her right to free counsel and would have to find and pay another lawyer. Actually, Waneta had already retained another attorney, Bill Sullivan, a renowned criminal defense lawyer and former district attorney from nearby Ithaca. Indeed, Sullivan was there in court, waiting for the green light. When he got it, he stepped in and convinced the judge to postpone sentencing for three months. "It appears that an innocent woman has been convicted of crimes she didn't commit, crimes that didn't happen," Sullivan said.[31]

Sullivan, who would later explain that he took the case without charge, made motion after motion to the court in what turned out to be a futile effort to further forestall sentencing and convince the court that Waneta merited a new trial. On September 11, Waneta was finally sentenced.

Having been convicted of five counts of murder, Waneta would have to spend at least 15 years in prison and could spend as much as the rest of her natural life behind bars. And that was only if the judge imposed the minimum sentences for each of the five convictions and ordered them to be served concurrently. In that case, Waneta would have been eligible for—but by no means guaranteed—parole in 15 years. The judge opted for the minimum sentence for each count—15 years to life—but directed that the sentences run consecutively, meaning that Waneta would not even be eligible for parole for 75 years. In effect, at age 49, she was given a sentence of life with no hope of parole.

Within days of her sentencing, Waneta was transported to Bedford Hills Correctional Facility, a women's prison just outside New York City and a long, hard drive from Owego. Not long afterward, I heard from Waneta's husband, Tim, who faithfully made that drive every week in an undependable car I would not have driven across town. Tim was upset because Waneta's physical condition appeared to be deteriorating rapidly, and prison officials were ignoring her medical problems. Having worked with inmates in New York prisons, including many women, over the years, I knew that Tim probably had good reason to be concerned about the care his wife was receiving—or, more appropriately, not receiving. Though my formal role in the case was long over, I agreed to contact the prison and use whatever clout I could muster to see that Waneta got the medical tests she appeared to need. Ultimately, the prison gave in and looked into Waneta's physical complaints, finally sending her to an outside medical facility where she was diagnosed with advanced pancreatic cancer.

Knowing that her life would soon be over, Waneta sought what the law calls "compassionate parole." She wanted to go home to die. In New York, a prison inmate in Waneta's condition was eligible for release. In Waneta's case, however, there was a hitch. Compassionate parole did not apply to any inmate convicted of murder. Thus, Waneta would have to die behind bars, a couple of hundred miles from her husband, son, and family.

On August 9, 1998, Waneta died. In one final bizarre twist, she was soon formally exonerated. Under New York law, since she died before her appeal had been heard, her conviction was vacated. As a result, the moment she died, Waneta Hoyt was no longer guilty of murder.

CHAPTER 2

Battered Woman Syndrome, Self-Defense, and Extreme Emotional Disturbance

2

As the author of several books and having testified in many high-profile trials over the past 30 years, I often receive letters and phone calls from people who are in trouble with the law and feel they or their cases could benefit from the intervention of a forensic psychologist. Almost all these letters and calls come from (or on behalf of) prison inmates who have been convicted of a crime and are seeking help in getting a new trial. Many of their stories are compelling, but rarely can I be of any assistance to them.

Sadly, for most people who call or write, it is too late. They might have fared better at trial if they'd had an evaluation by and testimony from a forensic psychologist. But by the time I hear from them, they have been convicted and their odds of having their convictions overturned and getting a new trial are somewhere between slim and none.

Once in awhile, however, I receive a call or a letter from someone I can help or at least try to help. That was the case when in early 1988 I received a short note from Charline Brundidge, who was then an inmate at the Monroe County Jail in Rochester, New York.

Charline wrote that she was a battered woman who killed her abusive husband and recently had been convicted of murder. She had read a newspaper article about my book *Battered Women Who Kill,* and wondered if I could look into her case. Ordinarily my answer would have been "no" but Charline added details that led me to at least consider further inquiry into her case.

I learned from the letter and from follow-up conversations with her attorney, John Speranza, that while Charline had been convicted, her conviction had been overturned under highly unusual circumstances, and she was awaiting a new trial.

A day after Charline's conviction, defense attorney John Speranza was in his office when he received an unexpected telephone call. The caller was the wife of one of the jurors who had heard the case against Charline and convicted her of murder. She told Speranza that she thought it "unfair" that her husband had been allowed to serve on the jury in a case involving allegations of spouse abuse since he had been abusing her for years.[1]

Though the caller may not have known the significance of what she was reporting, Speranza, a veteran criminal defense lawyer, recognized it immediately. He knew that as part of the extensive *voir dire* (attorney questioning of potential jurors), this woman's husband (like all members of the jury pool) had been asked whether he had ever been involved in any sort of family violence. Before being impaneled, he had replied "No."[2] Now, his wife was telling Speranza that he had beaten, choked, and threatened to kill her.

Soon after Charline's conviction, a hearing was held on Speranza's motion to set aside the verdict and order a new trial. The juror's wife testified that in 45 years of marriage she had called the local police 20 to 30 times to report assaults by her husband. Police records indicate that she filed three crime reports during those years but that her husband, the juror, was never charged. She testified further that her husband had last beaten her around the time of Charline's conviction, but had not harmed her since because she threatened him with a knife.[3]

The juror testified that he had answered "no" to the pretrial question about experience with family violence "Because it was never any physical violence against my wife. I was never arrested, never convicted and never went to court. Petty arguments go on all over the world."[4]

The juror did, however, acknowledge on cross-examination by Speranza that when he was questioned before trial he recalled at least one of the incidents in which his wife had called the police regarding alleged abuse. Speranza asked the juror, "As a result, did you say anything to the judge, myself or the prosecutor about your recollection?" "No," the juror replied.[5]

The prosecutor argued that the juror had not lied to the court because the question posed could have been interpreted as pertaining only to arrests for family-related violence. Moreover, the prosecutor argued that, even if the juror had lied, he "did not conceal facts, bias or prejudice which would have disqualified" him from serving on the jury in this case—one in which the defendant's defense of extreme emotional disturbance rested largely on her claim that she had been repeatedly and brutally abused by the man she killed.[6]

The judge made it clear early on in the proceedings that he wasn't buying those arguments. In response to the juror's testimony he said: "I very clearly asked about accusations of family violence. It's inconceivable to me how anybody could misinterpret the question and statement that was given to the jury panel."[7] To the publicly expressed disappointment of the prosecutor, the judge ruled that the juror's failure to disclose the allegations of abuse made against him by his wife denied Charline a fair trial. As he wrote in his 12-page decision, "It is difficult for the court to determine how [the juror] could have separated his own experiences, including the accusations of spousal abuse by his wife, from an objective assessment of the defendant's credibility."[8] The prosecutor appealed the judge's order, and the appeals court affirmed that order, setting the stage for a new trial.[9]

After learning these details, I agreed to examine Charline with regard to extreme emotional disturbance, which was raised in the initial trial, but also *battered woman syndrome,* which hadn't been considered. Since Charline was incarcerated and indigent, I agreed to conduct the evaluation and, if warranted, testify in her second trial without charge.

If I found that Charline had killed her husband while in a state of extreme emotional disturbance for which there was a reasonable cause or explanation and testified to that finding, that evidence might be sufficient for a jury to find her guilty of manslaughter rather than murder. However, if I found that she suffered from battered woman syndrome and, as a result, reasonably feared imminent death or serious bodily injury at the time she shot and killed her husband, that conclusion might be sufficient to allow the jury to acquit her on grounds of self-defense.

Psychological testimony is not usually involved in self-defense cases, and when it is, it is almost always involved in support of the self-defense claim of a battered woman or battered child who has killed his or her abuser.

The legal test of self-defense is whether the defendant reasonably believed that she was in imminent danger of being killed or seriously injured. This is both a subjective and an objective test. The defendant must have actually believed that she was in imminent danger of being killed or seriously injured, and that belief must have been reasonable.

Most of the time when self-defense is raised as a defense to homicide charges, there has been a killing during some kind of confrontation, during which the decedent threatened the defendant and the defendant responded with deadly force. At least that's generally the story that the defendant tells.

The jury then has to decide: first, whether to believe the defendant's description of what happened; second, whether the defendant, under those circumstances, actually did feel threatened; and third, whether a reasonable person would have felt threatened under those circumstances.

As I like to tell my law students, the reasonable person is the person on the jury, who is really saying to himself or herself, "Would

I have been afraid of being killed or seriously injured if it had been me in that situation?"

Generally there is no need for psychological expertise in these cases because a lay jury is capable of understanding the issues and judging for themselves whether the defendant acted in self-defense.

A problem for most battered women who kill their abusers is that most do not do so during a confrontation or abusive incident. Understandably, given the dynamics of battering relationships, many if not most battered women who kill their abusers do so while the batterer is asleep or otherwise preoccupied.

Thus the battered woman homicide defendant starts out with a major strike against her: the killing does not look like self-defense as most people envision that legal concept. As I detailed in *Battered Women Who Kill*—the book that Charline Brundidge had read about before contacting me—I did a study of 100 cases in which battered women killed their abusers. In these cases, the vast majority of the women killed their batterers not during a battering incident, when their fear of death or serious bodily injury might well have appeared reasonable, but rather sometime after a battering incident. Only about a third of these women killed their batterers while the batterers were physically attacking them. The remaining two-thirds killed their batterers after being physically battered or verbally abused. Significantly, in about 18 of these cases, the killing took place while the batterer was asleep or nearly asleep.[10]

In these cases, with nothing more than the woman's stated fear of death or serious bodily injury, conviction is almost assured because the jury will have an extremely difficult time finding that the woman's perception of danger was reasonable. After all, they will probably reason, "What danger does a sleeping man pose?"

Beyond that issue, however, battered women who claim self-defense as a justification for killing their abusers are often met with a host of other obstacles to acquittal, not the least of which are stereotypes and myths about battered women that lead jurors to doubt their claims that they were severely abused and that they honestly and reasonably feared death when they killed their abusers.

Psychological research provides the basis for a psychologist or other mental health professional to examine the battered woman defendant and, where appropriate, to offer expert testimony on her situation.

In most cases, the expert testimony sought to be introduced in these trials describes the battered woman syndrome, a pattern of physical and psychological abuse inflicted on a woman by a man with whom she shares an intimate relationship.

Dr. Lenore Walker (who coined the term) and others have written extensively about the syndrome, which among other things explains the psychological, social, and economic forces that prevent a battered woman from leaving her batterer.[11]

Although some courts have ruled that expert testimony on the battered woman syndrome is irrelevant to the battered woman homicide defendant's claim of self-defense and thus inadmissible, most have admitted such testimony on the theory that it bears on a crucial issue of fact "beyond the ken" of the average lay jury.

As the New Jersey Supreme Court explained in the seminal case of *State v. Kelly:*

> The crucial issue of fact on which this . . . testimony would bear is why, given such allegedly severe and constant beatings [the] defendant had not long ago left decedent. [C]ommon knowledge tells us that most of us, including the ordinary juror, would ask himself or herself just such a question. And our knowledge is bolstered by the expert's knowledge, for experts point out that one of the common myths, apparently believed by most people, is that battered wives are free to leave[,] that the battered wife is masochistic [and] that the "beatings" could not have been too bad for if they had been, she certainly would have left. The expert could clear up these myths.[12]

That is a pretty good description of at least part of the relevance of expert testimony in these battered women homicide cases, but there is usually quite a bit more.

In many cases, where appropriate, based on the expert's evaluation of the woman, the expert can explain to the jury why, despite the fact that the batterer was not beating the woman at the moment of the killing, the woman nevertheless feared that if she did not kill him, she would be killed or seriously injured.

The expert may also be able to explain how the woman's fear was reasonable (1) because battered women live in a continuous state of fear; (2) because, as a result of experience with the batterer over time, battered women learn to "read" their batterers and to predict the level of abuse they are about to suffer; and (3) because research and clinical experience with battered women indicate that many battered women are in fact killed or seriously injured by their batterers and that the danger of death or serious bodily injury to a battered woman is greatest any time she makes any effort to control the relationship or leave the relationship.

Charline had killed her husband, Marvin Brundidge, by shooting him five times while he was lying on a bed engaged in a telephone conversation with the local 911 operator. As a tape of the 911 call indicated, Marvin had placed the call and asked to have the police sent to the couple's home because "My wife is leaving and I don't want her coming back. I just want them to be here if she comes back."[13] On the tape, Marvin's request was followed by five gunshots and then Charline telling the operator she had just shot her husband.

The shooting followed an altercation between Charline and Marvin and there was little question that she may have been emotionally disturbed at the time. As for self-defense, however, it did not appear at first blush that Charline had killed her husband out of fear of imminent death or serious bodily injury, especially since he was on the telephone at the time, calling the police ostensibly to make sure that she left the house and stayed away from him.

As I began to evaluate Charline, I was skeptical, as I always am in examining a criminal defendant. But over the hours, as I listened to Charline's story of her life, including the abuse she had suffered at the hands of Marvin, reviewed hospital records of her injuries, and spoke to relatives who corroborated portions of her story, my skepticism diminished and I eventually became convinced not only that she was a battered woman but that she had, in fact, killed Marvin in self-defense.

At trial, over the prosecutor's strenuous and repeated objections, I was given extraordinary latitude in relating Charline's life story to the jury. The prosecutor, Charles Siragusa, was understandably distraught by the judge's decision in this regard, as my testimony obviated the need to have Charline testify in her own behalf, as she had done in the first trial. Thus, the jury would hear Charline's story from beginning to end, and Siragusa would have no chance to cross-examine her as he had done in the earlier proceeding.

Prior to giving Charline's story, I explained to the jury what is meant by battered woman syndrome. The following is an abbreviated version of what I said, with the dozens of objections raised by Siragusa redacted:

> Well, as I said, [battered woman syndrome] encompasses the type of abuse and how the abuse occurs. Generally what we found related to this syndrome is that women who are physically abused are also mentally abused.... [M]any of them are also sexually abused ... forced to have sex against their will by their batterers....
>
> The other thing that [battered woman syndrome] encompasses in terms of describing the nature of the abuse is that we've learned in studying the syndrome that batterers don't beat women 24 hours a day 365 days a year. The beatings ... are generally unpredictable. They occur at random times but follow a pattern, a cycle of violence....
>
> Almost invariably in battered woman syndrome ... there are three stages to the abuse. The first is a tension building stage where there is a lot of psychological abuse, name calling, minor kinds of physical abuse, pinching, poking, maybe pulling hair, slapping, that sort of thing and that eventually, the tension reached the point where there's an out and out battering incident where the man actually beats the woman physically. That's the second stage is the beating, and it's followed almost invariably by a third stage and that third stage we call contrition. It's a stage where the batterer becomes contrite, apologetic, oh I'll never do that again. I'm sorry, I didn't mean it. Please don't leave me. Please stay with me. Give me another chance, and that's particularly important because we found that these, the cycle of violence always ends on a positive note. It always ends with the batterer saying it won't happen again and giving the woman an incentive to stay in the relationship....

Two things related to how the woman feels and how she reacts . . . are critical. One is you almost always see social isolation in these cases. . . .

It varies but what it always means is that the batterer makes efforts to keep the woman in tow. The batterer may spy on the woman, may follow the woman, may insist that the woman account for her whereabouts at all times, constantly accusing the woman of infidelity to try to keep her in line. Also things like not allowing the woman to have friends in the home. Very important. The idea generally seems to be that if you do not let the woman have friends in the home then people won't find out what actually goes on behind closed doors. It can take other forms. Sometimes it takes the form of threats. Don't tell people I did this to you. Don't talk about our relationship with other people. I saw you talking with that guy. You must have been talking about us. . . .

[It is] almost. . . . like a pathological jealousy. I want to own you. I want to possess you. . . .

We always find efforts, coupled with this effort to socially isolate the woman, efforts to tear down her self-esteem. You're no good. You're rotten. You're vile. You're ugly, all sorts of expletives, ugly names with apparently one thing in mind. Make this woman feel so bad about herself that she won't leave because she'll have nowhere to go. She'll really believe that she is no good . . . that nobody else would have [her]. Why not leave? Well, part of the answer why not leave is because who would have me? I'm so awful. He's been telling me that for so long. . . .

There's several effects. To answer your question specifically, some battered women do reveal the abuse, some don't, and a lot of whether they reveal the abuse depends on the availability of people to reveal it to. If they have close family nearby or friends that they can reveal it to, they're more likely to. If they don't, they're less likely to. Of course, the other thing that plays a role in whether or not they reveal is what response they get from people when they reveal that they have been abused. . . .

[G]enerally the response that battered women get when they reveal the fact that they're abused is very negative. . . . The research indicates that battered women who reveal the facts that they're battered to relatives and friends are generally met with one or two kinds of responses. One, it can't be that bad because you are staying with him. Two, go back, make it work out. You love him. He loves you. You've got children. You have a family. You want to stay together. Save your marriage. The research also shows that women get a similar kind of response from the police . . . and from medical professionals, and outside of friends and family the two groups of people that battering comes to the attention of most are police, if they get called, and emergency room personnel. . . .

I worked in an emergency room. I saw a lot of battered women in an emergency room and the research really rings true for me. The research shows that battered women . . . come into an emergency room for physical injury and generally the response that they get is simply patch them up and send them out. The number one remedy that's given to battered women in emergency rooms in the United States is tranquilizing drugs, prescriptions for tranquilizers.

[The] initial response [of battered women to their abuse] is loss of self-esteem; feelings of worthlessness; feelings that the woman is no good, has nothing to offer; depression, feelings that she's depressed; feelings that she's helpless; feeling hopeless. It's called learned helplessness . . . [which] refers to what you see with battered women when they reach the point in the battering relationship where they really feel like nothing they do can make any difference, that they really can't change the situation, they can't get out of the situation. They reconcile themselves to, they sort of see it as their fate. . . .

[T]he typically battered woman like anybody in that type of situation, you try to minimize the abuse. Battered women develop strategies for appeasing their batterers, preventing them from battering them. Sometimes it's something as simple as, I know that "x" angers my husband so I won't do "x." Sometimes it's something as simple as knowing that when he comes home in a certain mood that's your signal to go in the other room or to suddenly have to go to the grocery store or to do something to get yourself out of the line of fire. You develop strategies for survival. . . .

[O]ver the course of a battering relationship, particularly a lengthy one, I mean, one that goes on over several years or more, as you would expect and as we've documented from the research, battered women reach the point where they can pretty much read the batterer. They have some idea of when he's going to strike, when a battering incident is going to happen. . . . They feel it coming and they get to the point where they can not only predict that the battering is coming but they have a pretty good idea of what the battering is going to be, how bad it's going to be. . . .

> One of the things that seems to differentiate battered women who kill from battered women who don't kill is [that] the women who kill are abused for longer periods of time. The women who kill are older generally than the women who don't kill. The batterers in those situations where the killing occurs have generally inflicted more serious abuse over a longer period of time, have generally also sexually abused the woman, and the fact that stands out in my own research is that invariably in the homicide cases . . . the batterer owns and uses a gun and the batterer is an alcohol abuser. . . .
>
> To me that's the deadly mix. You have an abuser who abuses a woman[,] who has a gun and who abuses alcohol and that seems, those three elements to spell death for either woman or the man.[14]

Following this general overview of the battered woman syndrome, I was permitted to detail Charline's life in describing the basis for my opinion. Again, deleting the dozens of objections made by Siragusa, the prosecutor, the following is a substantially abbreviated version of what I told the jury:

> Well, to begin with she was raped, sexually abused and beaten as a child. She has a classic victim childhood that you see in the battered woman syndrome. She was beaten by her mother with a belt repeatedly until she was 13 or 14 years old. She observed constant violence in her home, her parents beating each other with pots, pans, fists, knives. She was sexually abused by a neighbor when she was 11 or 12 years old. The neighbor broke into her house and she awakened to find the neighbor with his finger in her vagina. She was raped by a boy named Teodore when she was in the tenth or eleventh grade. He forced her to have sex. She became pregnant and she was raped by another young man, Edward . . . , whom she then married. He knew she was pregnant and knew that he wasn't the father of the baby. She married him. She returned to high school at the age of nineteen having dropped out to have her daughter and was raped by . . . a teacher who offered her a ride home, took her to a wooded area, chased her, forced her into the back seat, penetrated her vaginally then broke into tears and apologized for what he'd done and asked her not to say anything about it. . . .

Prior to her relationship with Marvin Brundidge, she showed what is again the classic battered woman syndrome adulthood. She was married, first of all, as a teen to Edward. . . . She lived with him on and off for five years. As I said before, he raped her the first time he had intercourse with her. He constantly put her down verbally. He slapped her around in front of his own family. He once threatened her with a gun. He was jealous. He followed her in a car, he had other people follow her. He kept her under surveillance. She finally got away from him after in front of their then baby Tyra . . . [he] choked her. At that point, Charline left under the guise of going to L.A., to Los Angeles, to set up a household for her and [Edward]. She got to Los Angeles and then she told him that she wanted a divorce, and at that point he had impregnated another woman and he had no objections to the divorce. . . .

Shortly thereafter, she embarked on another relationship in which she was abused. This was a relationship in which she went to Mexico, married a man named Arnold. She stayed with him for about three months, during which time he didn't beat her but he psychologically abused her and their relationship ended when she refused to have sex with him. He pinned her down, choked her, and tried to suffocate her by holding her nose and mouth shut. She begged for her life and he let her go.

The next relationship in this series [was with] a man named Adolph. . . . She dated him, never married him. He did not beat her but their relationship ended when he put a gun to her head . . . or chest in a parking lot. . . .

After leaving [Adolph], she embarked on a relationship where she dated Robert. . . . They fought frequently and she left him after he beat her up after a concert. As I say, that's what led up to the time of the relationship with Marvin. . . .

She . . . met Marvin by arrangement. Her sister and brother-in-law had arranged to have her meet Marvin, had told her that Marvin was looking for a woman, and Charline met him for the first time in New Jersey in July of 1978. They flew to Rochester and he put her up in The Americana Hotel. She spent about eight days there. . . . In the hotel, Marvin seemed to be a fun-loving person. She had a good stay with him during those eight days. He asked her not to leave him and promised to marry her the next month as soon as his divorce was finalized. He talked her into going to Los Angeles and quitting her job with the Los Angeles Police Department and then returning to Rochester. She did that . . . burned her bridges there, came back to Rochester, and was told by Marvin that he was getting back together with his wife, Fern, and Charline took a job at the University of Rochester. What I think is significant in terms of the syndrome here is that Marvin from September to February lived in and out of Charline's home. Sometimes he lived with her, sometimes he lived with his wife, but she tolerated that. She stayed with him despite the fact that he'd broken his promise, despite the fact that he was living part-time with Fern. She stayed for two reasons. She said she loved him and she'd burned her bridges behind her. She had nowhere to go. She'd given up her job, friends and life in California.

During these months, that September to February, Marvin occasionally slapped Charline, mostly in arguments over his relationship with Fern. There was one incident in which he accused her of dancing too close to a white man [both Charline and Marvin were black]. She denied it and he bit her face. . . .

May of 1979, he again confronted her with dancing, about dancing with another man. He said she knew who the man was. She said she didn't know who the man was. He said she was lying. He held her hands behind her back in the parking lot and punched her face until it was bloody. Charline then went to St. Mary's Hospital and had sutures for a cut on her chin and lip.

June, 1979, a month later, Marvin finally said, all right, I'm home to stay meaning he was back with Charline to stay. . . .

In December of '79 Marvin and Charline were married.

From January to December 1980, they had a fairly good relationship, what might be called a honeymoon period. There was one incident of abuse during early 1980. Marvin was jealous he said because Charline was talking to a Vietnam veteran in a bar. He called her aside. He took her outside. He shook her, slapped her, knocked her down into the snow, and when she got up knocked her down again. When she got up the third time, he grabbed her shoulders and bit her nose. . . .

January 1981, Fern, Marvin's ex-wife, her friend Sherry and a man named Doug came to Marvin's bar. Charline introduced herself as Marvin's wife and Marvin said, shit I don't got no wife. A while later Fern said something to Marvin and Marvin came over to Charline and hit Charline in the face . . . left the bar . . . and . . . came home to Charline three days later.

The same month, Marvin and Charline argued in a bar one night. Charline went home and put Marvin's clothes outside the door. Marvin came home, found Charline asleep, and then dragged her naked out of bed and into the kitchen area. He called her a bitch. He said, you bitch, you don't know who you're fucking with. He took out a knife from a drawer. He held it to her throat and told her he was going to kill her. Her daughter Tyra was there. . . . She saw it and pleaded with Marvin not to kill her mother. . . .

Later that same winter, Marvin accused Charline of flirting with a stranger. He took her in the backroom of the bar, threw her down into a cleaning bucket, injured her back. Then he held her down and beat her on the face with his hands and fist. At this time Charline called the police. She told them she'd been assaulted. She told them Marvin did it. They arrested Marvin and Charline went to St. Mary's emergency room and was treated there. . . .

Marvin was home that very night. He'd been arrested. They told Charline to go to the emergency room. She gets home and Marvin comes home that very night and talked her out of pressing charges. So, she dropped the charges against him. . . .

Around Thanksgiving, actually before Thanksgiving, excuse me. November 5, this is Charline's birthday. [T]hey were arguing in a car. Marvin spit at her. She spit back. He got out of the car on the I-390 and pulled her out of the car bodily, slapped her and threatened to beat her up and make her walk home. She begged him not to leave her there. He didn't. He took her back to the apartment and she left and spent the night in a motel on Jefferson Road. The next day Marvin acted as if everything was okay and he asked her to go to a party with him.

During that time period, and I don't have an exact date on this, Marvin threatened Charline with a gun, put a gun to her and said, if you don't tell me what you've been doing, I'll blow your fucking brains out.

Around Thanksgiving time, he dragged Charline out of her sister's home bodily and this was after he wanted her to go to his son's house and she refused. So he dragged her out of the house bodily.

> In 1982, again, things were in this tension building stage. There was a lot of psychological abuse, a lot of verbal abuse, minor physical abuse until late in the year, again, around the holidays. . . .
>
> From that period on . . . he started to abuse her physically pretty much every weekend, slapping her, hitting her, beating her, constantly accusing her of infidelity, but at the same time hinting to her that he was having affairs with other women. Marvin did things like come to Charline's place of work and told her repeatedly, I'm going to catch you with your nigger. He laughed at her. He put her down. He constantly called her Puerto Rican, Indian, slut, whore, all sorts of vile names. He frequently told her that he would kill her, that he would fuck her up, that he would punish her, that he would make her suffer. He also sexually abused her during that period of time from 1983 until the time of his death. He became rough in his sex. He would tell her that he had to be rough with her sexually to punish her. At one time, he brought a white woman into their home at night and forced her to have sex, for Charline to have sex with him in front of this woman and then had sex with this woman in front of Charline in the same bed. He regularly forced himself upon her sexually. . . .
>
> He tried to socially isolate her. He wouldn't allow her to have any friends. He made her report to him every day after work from her job by 4:30 at the bar or you better explain where you were in detail. He always had to know where she was and what she was doing. She had to keep an almost hourly record for him to account for her whereabouts and then there's her own reaction. . . .
>
> Her reaction is typical of battered woman syndrome. She became depressed. She felt hopeless and helpless. She said, I have nowhere to go. Who am I going to turn to? People know. People have seen Marvin beat me in public and nobody does anything. I've talked to my mother and my mother said, what's the matter, Charline, you can't take a few licks?[15]

Asked the basis for my opinion that at the time she killed Marvin, Charline's mental state was such that she believed that she was in imminent danger of being seriously injured or killed, I explained as follows:

> As I said before, from 1983 until about the time of the killing, the physical abuse in this relationship was escalating in intensity and frequency. Marvin was slapping Charline all the time. In May of 1983 there was

an argument. He picked up a dishcloth, wrapped it around her head, and tried to choke her with it, stuck it in her mouth. He started throwing her clothes around. He hit her in the face with a coat hanger and grabbed her by the arm and told her to get the fuck out of this house right now. Marvin then called the police, and before the police arrived, he grabbed her—excuse me—just before the police arrived she grabbed him in the groin area and scratched him and that put an end to that altercation. The police quieted them down, told them both to work things out for themselves.

Later Tyra and Tyra's husband picked Charline up and they went to Marvin's bar. At the bar, another woman told Marvin that Charline had slammed the ladies room door. Charline denied it and there was an argument. Marvin took Charline outside. She came back into the bar to get her purse and then at this point she was assaulted, beaten by Marvin's son Rod while Marvin stood and watched. Rod choked her. He picked her up against the wall. He punched her in the side of the head near the eye. . . .

Charline went home and called the police and wanted to have Rod charged. Marvin came home, argued with her in front of the police, and talked her out of charging Rod with assault. Marvin said if she pressed charges against Rod he would press charges against her and it was at that point the police advised her to go to St. Mary's hospital, which she did.

Later in this incident, Tyra confronted Rod about hitting her mother and Marvin told Tyra, shut up or I'll let Rod do the same to you. . . . There was a family picnic that day. Charline threatened to tell members of the family what had happened. Marvin threatened her and warned her not to say anything to anyone that Rod had done the damage to her face. Later Rod apologized and even Marvin apologized, told her he was sorry, said, do you want a divorce. They actually made an appointment with a lawyer at that point to discuss it but Marvin talked Charline out of it telling her that, look, we can work it out. I love you. I care for you.

In June '83 . . . Charline revealed a lot of the abuse to members of her family. Her relatives uniformly when they heard what happened, they advised her to go back to Marvin and make things work out with him. . . .

Beginning in September, 1984, there were [*sic*] incident after incident in which Marvin threatened Charline, grabbed her, slapped her. He was constantly flying off the handle, hitting her for no reason at all.

His physical abuse became at this point unpredictable and almost random. There was nothing that she could do to even tell when it was going to happen. He would just fly off into rages.

By the beginning of April, Charline was feeling totally out of control, that she had no control of her life. Marvin was drinking heavily, abusing alcohol and abusing her more frequently. As she put it, I was on my Ps and Qs trying not to say or do anything that would trigger a beating. She also tried hard not to drink during that period because it seemed to her that every time she drank, that was the time when Marvin would beat her. Meanwhile, Marvin is constantly telling her to drink. They go out and she doesn't want to drink. He tells her she should drink. In early April, Charline is sensing that something really bad is happening, that the relationship is really, really getting bad. She feels that something terrible is going to happen to her but she feels trapped. She feels like there's no way out. She's telling herself she can handle it but at the same time saying, no I really can't handle it.

Two weeks before the killing, April 5 and 6, Charline went to Kelly's bar to try to get away from Marvin. Marvin came to the bar. He found her and started questioning about where she had been: Who were you with? What happened? He started drinking heavily. He took her home. He threw her on the sofa and he did something he hadn't done before. He spanked her as if she was a child.

Two weeks later, the day of the killing, they went out to the store to buy Marvin a new suit of clothes. Marvin gets very angry at Charline. Why? Because she suggested that he try the suit on with a pair of shoes in the store. He snaps at her. He yells at her. He denounces her in the store. They visited Tyra's house briefly and then they went drinking. They went to a number of bars. During the course of this, this is the afternoon and leading up to the evening of the killing, they're driving along. They see a man. Marvin says that man owes Archie [Marvin's brother] money. He gets out of the car, walks up and starts pointing at the man and comes back and tells Charline that this man is going to pay the money. He's very angry. Then they went to a series of bars, the Shantelle Lounge, the Elks Lounge, the High Hat. The High Hat is a bar owned by a man named Jimmy White. This is the same Jimmy White that Marvin has constantly accused Charline of having an affair with. . . .

What seems to have set this whole lethal chain of events that night off was this situation in Jimmy White's bar, the High Hat. Marvin is accusing her of having an affair with Jimmy White. . . . They leave the bar. They get in the car and Marvin tells Charline, I know you're fucking Jimmy White. I'll kill you if I ever catch you and later on the way home Marvin tells Charline he has all the evidence he needs. I know you're fucking Jimmy White so I'm going to kill you. Charline tried to talk him down. She asked him why he was always saying she was a whore, why she had to be the pig, why she had to be the slut, why he always said she was fucking around when he's the one who apparently was unfaithful at least to her thinking. Marvin about a block away from the house becomes enraged. He gets a look on his face that Charline never sees before. His lips are quivering. His nostrils flare. His eyes are glassy. . . .

They get up to the house. Marvin stops the car. They get out. Marvin follows Charline up to the house. She goes to the bedroom to change out of what she called her good jumpsuit. She's undressing. Marvin comes in and puts his gun and holster—he carried a gun with him all the time. He carried it strapped to his ankle in a holster underneath his pant leg—puts his gun and holster in a chest of drawers. Charline thinks this is odd because every other night Marvin's routine has been to place that gun and holster on the nightstand beside the bed. . . . Then Marvin asks her repeatedly if she wants to fight with him. She says no, she doesn't want to fight and then he tells her, you better get out or I'm going to fuck you up, to use his words. . . . When she didn't move immediately, he grabbed her, choked her on the bed. She kicked him. He rolled off the bed. He grabbed her by the hair, pulled her off a chair and broke the chair. Then he picked her up and smashed her head into the wall. Charline looked at him and saw this hostile look that she'd seen before in the car. At this point she recalls Marvin saying, I'm going to fuck you up over and over. At that point he goes to the closet as if he's looking for something. Then he comes out and starts shadow boxing in the corner and pointing his finger at her. This is how she described it as if he had a gun in his hand and he was shooting. He then continues to tell her, I'm going to fuck you up. He picks up the phone and tells her wait right there, when I get off the phone you'll see. Wait till [*sic*] I get off the phone. She doesn't recall being aware of what he said on the phone other than his name.

> All of a sudden she found herself at the dresser. She had the gun out, and once she had the gun, her only thought was this is crazy, but then she thought at this point he's threatened her with death. She's pulled the gun on him. She's dead or he's dead. She shot him once and he grabbed the gun and then she fired more shots . . . and put the gun back in the drawer.[16]

Speranza then clarified that I knew that when Charline shot Marvin, he was on the bed talking on the telephone, and asked "Does that fact . . . alter or affect your opinion that Charline was in reasonable fear of imminent death or serious bodily injury when she shot the deceased?"[17] I replied "No, it doesn't at all" and then went on to explain why:

> You have to look at the whole thing in the context of what's gone on. First of all, this is a battered woman as a result of her experience being battered then for five or six years. She's able to read [Marvin] pretty well. She knows what's going to happen. She knows what he's just done to her. She knows what he's said: I'm going to kill you. I've got the evidence that you were fucking Jimmy White. I'm going to kill you.[18]

Siragusa's cross-examination was longer and more tedious than most—it went on for several days and consumed almost 300 pages of transcript—but was about what I had come to expect over the years of testifying in cases such as this one. He appeared especially frustrated, indeed angered—and I could not blame him—because he had been expecting a simple replay on the first trial. Not only was he hit with my testimony, but there was no need for Speranza to call Charline to the witness stand and expose her to cross-examination because the judge had given me virtual *carte blanche* to tell her story as I explained the basis for my expert opinions. Unable to cross-examine the defendant as he had planned, the only way Siragusa could attack Charline's account was by attacking me.

The bulk of Siragusa's attack was to repeatedly remind the jury, through questions to me, that I am a lawyer in addition to being a forensic psychologist. It seemed obvious to me that he wanted to take every opportunity to paint me as an advocate for Charline rather than a dispassionate, objective expert. He also brought up a number of other cases in which I had testified on behalf of defendants who had committed dreadful crimes, including child murder and molestation. The message he seemed to want to send the jury was that I was not only an advocate but an advocate for very bad people. He quizzed me about a job I had quit years earlier, a course he falsely stated that I had refused to teach, and how many subjects I had personally interviewed in my study of battered women who kill. Here it seemed that he was trying to paint me as somehow lazy or perhaps even incompetent.

The prosecutor also tried repeatedly to chip away at my testimony by citing minor inconsistencies between what Charline told me and what she had said to others. One of the peculiarities of this trial was that everyone in the courtroom, probably including most of the jurors, knew that Charline had been convicted of murder and granted a new trial, and that this was her second trail. But to avoid prejudicing the jury, we were explicitly required by the court not to refer to the previous trial. Thus, I often had to speak of learning certain facts from the transcript of a "prior proceeding." At one point, in his effort to point out inconsistencies, Siragusa slipped and asked me about something Charline said in "the last trial."[19] That question led to a motion for a mistrial, which was denied by the judge but could easily have been granted, thereby resulting in a third trial.

Siragusa also tried repeatedly to minimize Charline's injuries and to paint her as someone who really did not fit the generally accepted description of a battered woman. He pointed out, for example, that she had a job, had a credit card, and sometimes visited family, implying that these facts undermined my conclusion that she was a battered woman. For the most part, I was patient with the prosecutor, knowing that he was just doing his job, but at one point I could not help but turn the tables on him—becoming the questioner rather than the questioned.

I had just testified about the incident in which Marvin stood by and watched as his son assaulted Charline in public. Siragusa's sarcastic reply was "As did her daughter, Tyra Carpenter, as did her husband—Tyra Carpenter, as did her husband Kevin Carpenter, as did a bar full of people: is that right?" My response was "Would you stand by and watch someone beat your wife up?"[20] In retrospect, I probably should not have said that, but even professionals have their limits. As it turned out, however, those 11 words seemed to mark a turning point in the cross-examination.

At that point the judge intervened and the following dialogue ensued:

> *The Court:* Please, gentlemen. If you want to argue, that's fine. I think the jury would like to hear some facts. So try it again, Mr. Siragusa.
>
> *Mr. Siragusa:* Judge, respectfully, I'm trying.
>
> *The Court:* Respectfully too, you ask a question, you'll get an answer and we're not going to have any more arguing or we're going to discontinue the cross-examination right now. Is that clear, Mr. Siragusa?
>
> *Mr. Siragusa:* Yes, judge, it is.[21]

From that point on, the cross-examination seemed to lose much of its steam and became largely a rehash of questions that had already been asked and answered.

Dr. Richard Ciccone, then an associate professor of psychiatry at the University of Rochester, was called by the prosecution in an apparent attempt to rebut my testimony that Charline suffered from battered woman syndrome. Ciccone, who has since become one of the nation's leading forensic psychiatrists and a highly respected academic, had examined Charline prior to her first trial regarding extreme emotional disturbance and had testified against her on that issue in that trial.

In this second trial, Ciccone opined that Charline did not suffer from battered woman syndrome, but his opinion was undercut by several factors. Foremost, he acknowledged that he had never examined Charline with regard to battered woman syndrome or considered it as an issue in his evaluation of her, and had only looked at the issue because the prosecutor told him it was to be raised in the second trial.

Moroever, though clearly an erudite psychiatrist, Ciccone admitted to having read only one book about battered woman syndrome. Not surprisingly, the book he said he'd read was the one I had written, *Battered Women Who Kill*. On cross-examination, defense attorney Speranza ran through the titles of about a dozen other books on the subject, volumes written by Lenore Walker and others much more knowledgeable on the subject than I was; Ciccone admitted that he had never read any of them.

Despite his openly admitted ignorance of the subject, his acknowledgment that he knew Charline had been abused by Marvin on many occasions, and his admission that he had never questioned Charline about the major elements of battered woman syndrome (e.g., learned helplessness, cycles of violence, or even depression), Ciccone explained why Charline was not a battered woman suffering from battered woman syndrome when she killed her abusive husband:

> In my opinion, she did not demonstrate passive or dependent behavior prior to that time. I could find no evidence that she was either financially or emotionally trapped. As opposed to other circumstances where the husband will threaten the wife or girlfriend if she leaves, her husband was asking her to leave, and the information and the telephone call to 911 indicated that he had asked her to leave and didn't want her to come back. . . .
>
> Again the definition is not precise but generally speaking most people accept the fact that in the battered woman syndrome the woman is trapped, she is not allowed to leave. The man will hunt her down, will hurt her, will kill her, and yet if she stays she's in imminent danger so she's stuck, she can't go and she can't stay. In this case, Mrs. Brundidge—Mr. Brundidge appeared to be telling Mrs. Brundidge to leave, to get out, and wanted the police to reinforce that. . . .
>
> People talk about the pattern of escalating violence begins slowly, then it builds up to enormous violence and then there's a honeymoon over a good period that follows it, and in this circumstance, the interaction between the two indicates that they had fights from time to time but there was no evidence that it followed the pattern of escalation of violence that had been written about by some writers.[22]

Speranza briefly cross-examined Ciccone, concluding by asking him about a recent local newspaper article in which the psychiatrist was featured:

Q: Okay. Now, Dr. Ciccone, were you the subject of a newspaper article in December of '87?

A: I was.

Q: You were, and that article was called "Psychiatrists in the Courtroom, Hired Guns"?

A: That was the headline.

Q: That was the headline and that article talked about you, didn't it?

A: Among other people, yes.

Q: And that article said you were a hired gun?

> *The Court:* All right, Mr. Speranza. We don't want to start reading newspapers in here, please.
>
> *Mr. Siragusa:* Objection.
>
> *The Court:* I know you're just going to say what the article said. We're not going to get into what the paper said.
>
> *Mr. Speranza:* Okay.

Q: Doctor, you testified that last year you made $50,000 paid by the county, right?

A: Yes, Mr. Speranza . . .

Q: Now, you have a vested interest in testifying for Mr. Siragusa and these other people that pay you all this money, don't you?

A: I try and do a credible job.

Q: I know. I know, but, you certainly have a terrific economic stake in it, don't you?

A: It's part of my livelihood, sure.[23]

Speranza's attack on Ciccone's financial interest in serving the prosecutor may have been somewhat unfair, since the money earned by the psychiatrist from the county was for work done not only for the district attorney, but the public defender and other assigned defense attorneys. Still, it did seem odd that, having never examined Charline regarding battered woman syndrome and apparently knowing very little about the syndrome, an experienced expert such as Ciccone would have put himself in the position to be attacked in this way.

In the final analysis, however, except for whatever harm may have been done to the psychiatrist's reputation or ego, Speranza's cross-examination of Ciccone apparently was of no consequence. The jury rejected Charline's claims of extreme emotional disturbance and self-defense, and convicted her of murder.

The judge, who had obviously heard all the evidence, including the testimony of the two experts, imposed the most lenient sentence available under the law, 15 years to life in prison. That meant that, technically, Charline would be eligible for parole consideration after serving 15 years. But those in the know realized that parole for a convicted murderer after serving only 15 years was extremely unlikely and that a more probable outcome, given the politics of parole in New York at that time, was that Charline would never be released.

Charline went off to prison and proved to be a model inmate. Behind bars, she earned a bachelor's degree and counseled other inmates. About seven years or so into her sentence, Charline came to the attention of Mary Lynch, a law professor running a clinic for students at Albany Law School. Professor Lynch and her crew of law students investigated Charline's case, her trials, and her prison conduct, and determined that she would be a good candidate for clemency from New York's governor.

Lynch and her students must have realized that the odds were against them. To begin with, no New York governor had ever granted clemency to a battered woman who had killed her husband and been convicted of murder. Also, prosecutor Siragusa's boss, Monroe County District Attorney Howard Relin was adamant that Charline serve her full sentence. "We've had 24 citizens of Monroe County who agreed unanimously that she was guilty of murder," the DA told the press. "She had one of the best attorneys in Monroe County, John Speranza. To suggest she was unjustly convicted just flies in the face of the evidence that was at the trial."[24]

Having already been involved in one successful and many more unsuccessful clemency applications by battered women who had killed their abusers, and on whose behalf I had testified in other states, I knew what Lynch and her students were up against and I did not expect them to succeed. But they never gave up, gathering every bit of evidence they could that would support their petition for clemency. Among other things, they asked me to reevaluate Charline and to report my findings in a letter to the governor.

After two-and-a-half years of hard work on the case, Lynch and her students convinced New York Governor George Pataki to commute Charline's sentence to time-served.

In January 1997, after spending over a decade incarcerated, Charline Brundidge walked out of prison a free woman and began a new career counseling battered women. I don't know what role, if any, my testimony at her trial played in the ultimate decision in this case, but I was deeply touched and relieved when I read the *New York Times'* account of what influenced the governor to grant clemency to Charline. Buried in the middle of the page-one news story I read:

> Three letters to Mr. Pataki stand out in Ms. Brundidge's fat clemency file, which his wife read before inviting Ms. Lynch and her students to lunch at the Governor's Mansion, as a gesture of support.
>
> One is from Ms. Aycox [the former Tyra Carpenter], describing life before her mother's marriage. Despite being a single parent, Ms. Brundidge found time and money to take her to concerts, on trips and to elegant restaurants. She taught her to maintain good credit and be sure her purse and shoes matched.
>
> Another is from Charles P. Ewing, a professor of law and psychology and the author of a book about battered women who kill. His letter said he had never met anyone who made more effective use of incarceration. The third is from Ms. Brundidge's sentencing judge, Eugene W. Bergin, who told the Governor that hers was the only case he had seen in 32 years that merited commutation.[25]

CHAPTER 3

Insanity: Malingering versus Organic Brain Syndrome

3

Auburn, a small, formerly industrial city in central New York, has a rich history—at least in terms of the American criminal justice system. Auburn is widely known as the site of the Auburn Prison, New York State's first state penitentiary and the site of America's first execution by means of the electric chair. The penitentiary, a concrete and stone fortress, was built in 1816 as a model prison under what was then known as the "Auburn system." The Auburn system was a method of corrections in which inmates worked together in enforced silence in the daytime and were segregated in solitary confinement at night. To this day, the old Auburn Prison operates as the maximum-security Auburn Correctional Facility, part of New York's Department of Correctional Services, and it is probably the largest single employer in the Auburn area.

But Auburn is also well known for being the home of William H. Seward, who served as governor of New York, a United Sates senator, and secretary of state under President Abraham Lincoln. Though perhaps best known for his role in the 1867 purchase of Alaska (referred to by critics at the time as "Seward's folly" or "Seward's Icebox"), Seward was also an abolitionist and outspoken opponent of the Fugitive Slave Act, who, as an attorney, often defended runaway slaves.

In 1846, having served two terms as New York's governor and soon to embark on a successful campaign for the U.S. Senate, Seward put himself at the center of a raging controversy in Auburn. In two separates cases, Seward agreed to defend two African-Americans accused of murder. Henry Wyatt had allegedly stabbed to death a fellow inmate. William Freeman was accused of the stabbing deaths of four people he believed had falsely testified against him. Both men were mentally ill and had been brutalized while in prison. In the latter case, Seward raised one of the earliest insanity defenses in the United States, arguing, "Freeman is a demented idiot, made so by blows, which extinguished everything in his breast but a blind passion of revenge."[1] Both defendants were convicted, despite Seward's eloquent and zealous defenses. Wyatt was executed; Freeman died in prison awaiting an appeal of his conviction.

It would not be until 143 years later that Auburn would see another local insanity trial even close to the magnitude of the *Freeman* case: the 1989 murder prosecution of another African-American man, James Leo ("Jimmy Lee") Rouse.

On the evening of March 26, 1988, Jimmy Lee Rouse, a 29-year-old ex-convict went to Robie's Bar and Grill with friends who were celebrating an anniversary. Rouse had a couple of drinks before going to Robie's and consumed an undetermined quantity of alcohol at the bar prior to closing time. As the bar was closing, around 2 AM, Rouse got into an argument with another patron, John "Pete" Tillman. As Tillman was approaching Rouse's friends, Rouse muttered "Another one of them damn Tillman's" and pushed Tillman.[2] When Tillman replied, "You don't know me," another patron, Frederick Thomas, inserted himself between the two men.[3] Rouse responded by grabbing a barstool, throwing it through a plate glass window, and shouting "All you motherfuckers are dead" as he left the bar.[4]

On leaving the bar, Rouse spotted a car being driven by a woman he knew. Rouse pushed his way into the car, demanded to drive it and, against the woman's will, sped off with her in the front seat on the passenger side. After a short but erratic drive, during which Rouse drove the vehicle over an embankment, he stopped the car in the middle of a street, got out, and ran away.

Meanwhile the police had been summoned to Robie's, had taken a report of the altercation, and left. A short time later, as Tillman, Thomas, and bartender John Reddick were cleaning up the mess created by the damage to the window, Rouse returned to the bar armed with a 12-gauge shotgun. One of the men heard Rouse say, "My name is Jimmy Lee Rouse."[5] Another heard him shout, "Yeah, mother fuckers, I'm back."[6] Thomas threw up his arms and pleaded, "Mister, please don't shoot me, please don't shoot me."[7] Rouse cocked the gun and shot Thomas in the groin. Tillman tried to run but Rouse shot him in the chest. Rouse then fled the tavern, and Reddick used the telephone to summon the police. Both shooting victims were given emergency medical treatment. Thomas was seriously wounded but survived after a month-long hospitalization. Tillman died from blood loss shortly after he was shot.

Police officers searched for Rouse but were unsuccessful until about 4:45 PM, that day, when they found him at the home of his sister. Rouse surrendered, telling the arresting officers that he had been at Robie's the evening and early morning before, had become intoxicated, and was "jumped" by at least two other men. Rouse denied commandeering the car or shooting anyone but added that one of his attackers had struck him over the head with a beer bottle. He told the officers that the next thing he remembered was awakening in the bushes outside Robie's Bar and Grill.

Rouse had a minor cut behind his ear, scrapes on his forearms, and a laceration on the upper part of one of his buttocks. He attributed these injuries to the incident in which he said he had been jumped and asked officers to get him medical attention. Rouse was taken to a local hospital emergency room, where staff observed a small area of soft tissue swelling above his right ear and some scattered abrasions but no signs of serious injury. A skull x-ray was normal and the examining physician found Rouse to be neurologically intact.

Charged with murder, attempted murder, unauthorized use of a motor vehicle, and unlawful imprisonment, Rouse was remanded to the county jail to await trial, which was eventually scheduled to begin January 9, 1989. Meanwhile, Rouse's court-appointed attorney indicated that he might offer a plea of insanity and extreme emotional disturbance on his client's behalf. Defense counsel retained a psychiatrist, Dr. Barbara Miller, to examine Rouse and report her findings.

Miller examined Rouse on December 9, 1988, and referred him to Dr. Thomas Lazzaro, a clinical psychologist, for testing that was conducted on December 29, 1988, and January 2, 1989. Pressed to prepare a written report before trial, Miller chose to do so without the full benefit of Lazzaro's testing. Her report indicated that she found Rouse suffered from organic brain syndrome and that he was insane at the time of the shootings.

Not being sure that a psychiatric defense would be offered, the prosecutor, District Attorney Paul Carbonaro hedged his bets and waited until he saw Dr. Miller's report before retaining an expert of his own. I was the expert retained by the district attorney, and I examined Rouse on January 6, 1989, just a few days before the trial began. Although my evaluation was done at the proverbial last minute, I had plenty of time to conduct a thorough examination. What I was unable to do before trial began was to review all the documents I wanted to see before reaching a conclusion and writing a report. Since some of the documents I wanted to see did not become available to the district attorney until the trial began, I never completed a written report. Instead, I verbally conveyed my opinion that Rouse was malingering, was not insane, and did not suffer from an extreme emotional disturbance at the time of the shootings.

I later learned from the trial transcript that another reason for waiting to retain an expert may have been the prosecutor's expectation that the defendant would plead guilty. In the opening moments of the trial, both the prosecutor and defense attorney made it clear for the record that Rouse had been offered the chance to plead guilty to second-degree murder and that, in exchange for that plea, he would be sentenced only for that crime. In other words, if Rouse pleaded guilty, the maximum sentence he would face would be 25 years to life, whereas if he went to trial and was convicted on all counts he faced the possibility of a sentence in the 50-years-to-life range. Rouse, who by then had the benefit of Dr. Miller's report, rejected the plea offer and opted to proceed to trial, offering defenses of insanity and extreme emotional disturbance.

Aside from the expert testimony, the evidence in Rouse's trial was presented quickly and with little if any controversy. Though there was never any real doubt about it, the testimony of a number of witnesses established that Rouse had indeed shot the two victims, killing one and seriously wounding the other. And while the evidence was clear that Rouse had commandeered a car outside the bar, the judge found insufficient evidence to allow the jury to consider the charge that he had unlawfully imprisoned the driver when he drove away with her still in the vehicle.

Rouse did not testify. The only two witnesses called on his behalf were Dr. Miller, the psychiatrist, and Dr. Lazzaro, the psychologist.

After establishing her qualifications, Dr. Miller began her direct testimony by describing the history she obtained from Rouse. According to Miller, Rouse remembered little of his childhood. Thus, her recitation of his history began when he was about 15 years old and was committed to the State Agricultural and Industrial School at Industry, a state reformatory commonly referred to as "Industry." Miller indicated that Rouse told her that while at Industry on December 14, 1974, he and another inmate escaped, stole a car, and collided with a tractor-trailer. Rouse claimed that he suffered a significant head injury—"a severe skull fracture"[8]—in the crash and that one of his shoulders had to be "sewed back on."[9] Miller also testified that Rouse told her that he was unconscious for three to four months after the accident. Surprisingly, however, she also testified, "I think it was probably more like at the most 10 days because Mr. Rouse remembers waking up on his birthday [December 25]."[10]

According to Miller, Rouse claimed that after this head injury he experienced headaches, auditory hallucinations (voices telling him to kill himself), visual hallucinations (a little green man and pink dog), difficulty paying attention, and suicidal thoughts. Miller also testified that following his release from the reformatory, Rouse graduated from high school, attended a community college and a four-year college without graduating from either, married, divorced, and fathered two children. According to Rouse, Miller testified, after the divorce, he went through a period of heavy alcohol consumption and was sentenced to prison for stabbing another man. State Department of Correctional Service records indicated that Rouse was sentenced to serve from 2.33 to 10 years in prison for that offense, but was released on parole after serving 34 months.

As for her assessment of Rouse's mental status at the time of her examination, Miller told the jury:

> He showed memory impairment. He showed perceptual distortions of hallucinations. His thought content contained suicidal ideation, suspiciousness and delusions. He showed depression, depressed mood, markedly low self-esteem. Behavior showed signs of social withdrawal, impulsivity, obvious violence or we wouldn't all be here, poor judgment and alcohol problems. Also he was eating very poorly.[11]

The psychiatrist added:

> He hears a dull humming sound in his ears. I mean these are other hallucinations, not voices but other sounds that are around there and in his ears and his temple area. He hears a lot of sounds that he can't tell where they are coming from, which he describes as high-pitched sounds, zooming sounds and hums. [H]e also occasionally hears someone calling his name as if from a far off distance and that this has been so convincing to him that for a long time he used to turn to look to see where this was coming from. . . .
>
> He also reported distortions in his sense of taste perception in that he was experiencing a rotten, a taste his food consistently [had] that he described as like a rotten orange. . . .
>
> The explanation that Mr. Rouse arrived at about that is that he believed that somebody was putting something in his food for the purpose of killing him.[12]

As for a diagnosis of Rouse, Miller offered several. First she testified that he was mildly mentally retarded. Next she testified that he suffered from chronic organic brain syndrome: "a mental disease or defect that means that there has been an impairment, a significant impairment in brain structure and function that is of long standing."[13]

This disorder, Miller told the jury, stemmed from "repeated head trauma"[14] and was characterized by "an accentuation of previous long-standing characteristic traits of recurrent outbursts of aggression and rage out of proportion to the precipitating psychological circumstances or stressers [*sic*], suspiciousness, paranoid ideation, impulse and explosive behavior that is dangerous to others."[15]

After adding further diagnoses of organic personality disorder and depression, Miller opined that Rouse had been suffering from an acute organic brain syndrome when he shot his victims. Indeed, she went so far as to state, "I am absolutely certain in every degree of reasonable medical certainty that Mr. Rouse suffered from an acute organic brain syndrome, okay?"[16] As Miller explained:

> Now, there are two, there are two kinds of acute organic brain syndromes. . . . One is called idiosyncratic alcohol intoxication with blackout. The second is concussion with a 12-hour anterograde amnesia. Both or either I am certain happened. Whether it's both or exactly which one I can't be sure, but that he had an acute organic brain syndrome I am certain. . . .
>
> Alcohol idiosyncratic intoxication . . . is characterized by behavior that is atypical of the person's behavior when he's not drinking. It occurs after a small amount of alcohol ingestion that would not cause major alterations in behavior in most people.[17]

As for the diagnosis of concussion, Miller explained her reasoning as follows:

> One was Mr. Rouse's report of being hit on the head with a beer bottle, seeing a white flash and that's it, no memory. That's his report.
>
> Another piece of evidence that I had available to me was his visit to the . . . Emergency Room and their evaluation and a photo you showed me that was taken at that time that showed that he had a bump on his head. . . .
>
> The flash of light of that kind of acute is quite consistent. The memory loss, total memory loss from the time of the event is quite consistent and

> remember, right up until, by Mr. Rouse's account to me, right up until the time of the flash of light and the pain in his head, he was remembering as best as he perceived it. He was giving a detailed account of his memories of what proceeded. . . .
>
> Then all the other things, you know, not being able to be aware of what he's doing, not being able to plan, automatic pilot kind of behavior, all that stuff is consistent with the kind of things that a person who has a concussion may do.[18]

When I examined Rouse, I was extremely skeptical of his story, essentially the same one that he told Dr. Miller. But I was most doubtful of his claim that at the age of 15 he had suffered a skull fracture, been in a coma for a month, had both arms torn from his torso at the shoulder, and had to have them surgically reattached. At my request, Rouse had shown me his shoulders, and I observed no scarring or any other evidence that would indicate that he had undergone major orthopedic surgery.

His story to me about the coma and to Miller about being unconscious for weeks was not documented in any of the records I saw or she saw. I requested to see Rouse's records from Industry but the district attorney had been told that staff there could not locate them. I felt that those records might be critical in confirming or disproving Rouse's claim about the head injury, so I suggested that the district attorney check with a good friend of mine who lived in Auburn and worked for the state agency that operated the reformatory at Industry. My friend was able to get the staff at Industry to make another effort to look for Rouse's record. On the lunch break after Miller completed her direct testimony, the district attorney finally got the records.

The Industry records indicated that Rouse had indeed escaped with another youth and stolen a car, but was treated only briefly at a hospital for facial lacerations and then released and returned to the reformatory. There was no mention of a skull fracture, coma, or severed and surgically reattached arms. The records also indicated that a routine psychiatric evaluation conducted on December 28, 1974, two weeks after the car accident, found Rouse to be normal.

Confronted with this record on cross-examination, Miller (who had also seen it during the recess) belittled it as not being a medical record but only an institutional record, and implied that the failure to include specific reference to the injuries Rouse claimed did not mean that those injuries had not actually occurred.

Miller remained steadfast in defending her opinion, even as Carbonaro did his best to impeach her testimony with the record before her. After much back and forth, the district attorney finally got the psychiatrist to concede that Rouse must have deceived or misled her about the injuries he suffered in the 1974 crash, injuries that went to the heart of her diagnosis of chronic organic brain syndrome. As regards Rouse's claim to have had his arms severed, two questions were all that was needed:

Q: Doctor, if his arms were severed on December 14, it would have been impossible for him to have a normal psychiatric exam two weeks later; would it not?

A: First of all—

Q: Is that yes or no, Doctor?

A: Given the assumptions, if the assumptions in your question are accurate, the answer is yes.[19]

With regard to the alleged skull fracture and protracted coma, only one question was necessary:

Q: If the defendant suffered a severe skull fracture of the type he described to you and in fact was comatose for three to four months, it would have been impossible for him to have had this normal psychiatric evaluation on December 28, 1974, is that true? He wouldn't have been conscious?

A: That's correct. Yeah, that's correct.[20]

Despite these forced concessions, Miller insisted that the inconsistencies between Rouse's account and that contained in the record did not matter. For example:

Q: Let me ask you this, Doctor. The accuracy of your diagnosis is based on the truthfulness of the statements that were given to you by Jimmy Lee Rouse; isn't that right?

A: That is not true.

Q: If his statements were false to you, your opinion would not be accurate; is that true?

A: That is not true. . . .

Q: In other words, Doctor, what you said then is if James Rouse gave you an inaccurate medical picture of himself, that wouldn't change your opinion; is that true?

A: It does—I have to take that into account but it does not alter my conclusions as I stated them here today.[21]

When Miller defended her diagnosis based on Rouse's reports of three head injuries other than the claimed skull fracture alleged followed by coma, Carbonaro responded with a classic cross-examination ploy that Miller was unable to resist:

Q: Dr. Miller, if the defendant did not suffer a severe skull fracture as described to you in 1973, as a result of that accident, would that change your opinion?

A: First of all—

Q: Yes or no?

A: No, it would not change my opinion.

Q: Okay. If the defendant did not suffer an injury as he described to you in Cortland in 1981, would that change your opinion?

A: No.

Q: If the defendant did not suffer head trauma as he described to you by striking his head in the shower at Industry in 1974, would that change your opinion?

A: No.

Q: If the defendant did not suffer any organic brain trauma as a result of that alleged injury while incarcerated in prison in 1984, I believe you testified to in 1985, would that change your opinion?

A: No . . .

Q: So, if the defendant didn't suffer any of those four head traumas, your opinion would still be the same; is that true?

A: That's correct.[22]

Questioned next about her opinion that Rouse may have been suffering from idiosyncratic alcohol intoxication on the night of the shootings, Miller and Carbonaro engaged in the following exchange, which I found truly remarkable given the definition of idiosyncratic alcohol intoxication that Miller, herself, had given on direct examination:

A: As far as my basic opinion of idiosyncratic alcohol intoxication, if that condition can be caused by a couple of drinks, it certainly can be caused by multiple drinks. So it doesn't matter how many it was.

Q: So if he was extremely drunk, you are—

A: It only is that much more weight to my opinion.[23]

Finally, Carbonaro quizzed Miller on what he saw as the difference between a clinical evaluation and a forensic evaluation, a distinction that appeared to be lost on the general psychiatrist, who had handled only three other forensic cases in her career and had never before evaluated a murder defendant:

Q: Could you tell me please, would I be correct if I assume that you approached this evaluation differently than you do a regular evaluation in your everyday practice since this one—

A: No, you would not be correct in assuming that.

Q: Did you approach this one the same way you would as an evaluation you do in your office?

A: Absolutely . . .

Q: So you approached this evaluation the same as anyone in your office notwithstanding the fact that this person you interviewed was accused of murder?

A: I'm not sure I understand what you mean.

Q: You had the same frame of mind interviewing this person, Jimmy Lee Rouse, that you have when you interview other people in your office?

A: I think so.

Q: So you weren't any more careful even though this person was accused of murder?

A: Of course, I was extremely careful. I am always extremely careful.[24]

The second and only other witness for the defense was the psychologist, Dr. Lazzaro. Lazzaro testified very briefly that he had administered a number of psychological tests. Lazzaro testified that he believed that "Mr. Rouse does suffer organically based deficits," but he never said why.[25] Indeed, defense counsel then asked him why he had mentioned in his report, "The diagnostic categories generated by [Rouse's] MMPI [Minnesota Multiphasic Personality Inventory] profile include substance dependence, antisocial personality disorder and schizotypal personality disorder."[26] Lazzaro explained, "I offered those in that paragraph to Dr. Miller as rule-out diagnoses for her consideration. In other words, I was giving her information to consider in making her diagnostic determination, giving her those diagnoses to rule out based on her interview and other clinical data."[27]

After Lazzaro's testimony, I was called as a rebuttal witness. Here, as is often the case when testifying as an expert for the prosecution, I had a distinct advantage over my colleagues who testified on Rouse's behalf: I had the opportunity not only to read their reports but to hear their testimony before giving mine. Also by the time I testified, I felt quite confident that the district attorney had succeeded in undermining

Dr. Miller's opinion by demonstrating that Rouse had not been truthful with her.

After some background questions about my credentials and what I had done in the case, Paul Carbonaro immediately set about using my testimony to cast even further doubt on Dr. Miller's conclusions. First we tackled what Miller had described as "distortions in [Rouse's] sense of taste perception."[28] I explained to the jury:

> He told me that he had taste hallucinations and when I asked him what he meant by that, he said, well, I have a bad taste in my mouth when I eat; and I explored that with him and he explained to me that he has a very bad stomach problem, that he has to eat as many as five Rolaids every time after every meal and sometimes after even having a cup of coffee and that he gets a backup of what he said, he called bile. Apparently his stomach backs up into his throat and he gets a bad taste after he eats. That's what he said these, what he called the taste hallucinations were, a bad, bad aftertaste in his mouth from his stomach.[29]

Next Carbonaro asked me about Rouse's alleged auditory hallucinations and I explained that "[H]e referred to that as noise hallucinations, too, and I said, are you hearing this noise now that you referred to, and he said, yes. Since I could hear it too, I said, are you referring to the fan, the noise coming from the fan, and he said, yes, that's the noise I'm referring to."[30]

Following these discussions, we turned to my diagnoses: malingering and antisocial personality disorder.

As regards malingering, I told the jury:

> [M]alingering essentially refers to somebody who is pretending to be ill, and in this case I saw essentially seven categories of evidence to suggest that in the course of the evaluation I did with Jimmy Lee Rouse. The first has to do with his claim of amnesia. He claimed two amnesias. One is that he has total amnesia for his childhood up until the time he was 12 or 13 years old. He has absolutely no recollection of anything. The other amnesia he has, according to him, is for the events surrounding the shooting and the death for which he's charged. He claims that he was

hit with a beer bottle and that thereafter for 12 hours or thereabouts, he remembers absolutely nothing.

The first thing that I noted about that in terms of the malingering diagnosis is that this is an implausible combination of amnesias. It would be exceedingly rare to find someone with both this retrograde amnesia, this backward amnesia he claims from childhood, and then this anterograde or forward amnesia he claims from the beer bottle injury; but more than that, this combination of amnesia and his description of it does not fit any known pattern of amnesia.

Essentially what you have here is a guy who is claiming that he has amnesia for these events but all the medical tests indicate no organic basis. The electroencephalogram, EEG, tests, are negative. They say no organic problem. He had two neurological examinations done by a neurologist. They say no neurological problem.

In the absence of that, the amnesia he claims would have to be what we call functional amnesia or emotionally or psychologically based. For him to have a functional forward-looking amnesia, as he claims, is almost unheard of. I have never seen it in my practice and I can't find any documentation of it in the literature.

So his amnesia is the first thing that tells me he was malingering. It's simply false.

The second is a series of inconsistencies between what Mr. Rouse told me and what the documents show and what other people show. First, he claimed that he had a, he suffered a skull fracture in this accident at Industry.... He told me he definitely had a skull fracture, that he had seen the medical records at Industry and they definitely said skull fracture, that he had plastic surgery on his face, that he had serious physical injuries, he said that both of his arms had been severed from his body.

The records indicate that he suffered from facial lacerations, that he was treated and released from the hospital. That was December 14. It's not clear from the record exactly the date he was discharged but the memo that says that was dated December 17, so within three days of the accident he was back at Industry....

It's implausible to me as an expert, as a psychologist, that someone could suffer those kinds of injuries, be treated in three days and be back at the state school at Industry.

Additionally, the records consistently indicate, and there ... were four examinations, there are two neurological examinations and two EEG examinations, both indicate no demonstrable brain injury....

He also told me that he was unconscious for a long period of time following that accident, told Dr. Miller he was unconscious for three to four months.

Again the records indicate that he was back at Industry within three days of the accident and, indeed, that within two weeks of the accident he was interviewed at Industry by a psychiatrist. So he clearly was not unconscious for three to four months.

He also told me that until the incident with the ... tractor where he got involved in what has been described as a joyride with a tractor, that he had no prior criminal involvement, no delinquency, that this was his first brush with the law.

The records indicate that he had several brushes with the law, several acts of delinquency prior to that incident.

He told me that he could not imagine or envision acting in a violent manner toward anyone, and during the same interview he told me, I don't take any shit from anyone. If somebody hits me, they're done for.

I saw that as inconsistent.

He also told me that part of the reason he knew that he didn't have a gun that night was because his family members would not give him a gun because they know the kind of rages that he flies into since he was discharged from prison.

The final inconsistency was, he told me that he had escaped from the County Jail because, "I was bugging out. The noises were amplified. I had to get the fuck out before I did something," and yet, there's been testimony from a witness that Mr. Lee [*sic*] told him that he escaped from the jail "to get that dude so he can't testify against me."

... The complex of symptoms that Mr. Lee—or Mr. Rouse, James Lee Rouse, shows here, essentially he is talking about a rather sudden onset of psychotic symptoms. They don't fit any known classification of mental illness and they don't fit the developmental pattern for developing this kind of severe mental illness that he's claiming.

He has no prior history of psychiatric evaluation or treatment. This is somebody who suddenly has come up with a rather serious form of psychopathology if you believe him.

> The final thing that led me to the diagnosis of malingering is the fact that there is obvious motivation in this case to malinger.[31]

As for the diagnosis of antisocial personality disorder, I used the American Psychiatric Association's *Diagnostic and Statistical Manual of Mental Disorders* (then in the third-revised edition) as an outline for explaining this diagnosis:

> Well, for antisocial personality disorder, there are fairly specific criteria that are laid out in the diagnostic and statistical manual. Essentially they're broken down into three categories: Current age at least 18. Defendant is roughly 30 years of age so he fits that category.
>
> The evidence of conduct disorder with onset before age 15 as indicated by, and then there is a list and there has to be at least three of these indications present in a case.
>
> What I found present in this case was running away from home at least twice while living in a parental or parental-surrogate home; two, often initiated physical fights; three, deliberately destroyed others' property; four, deliberately engaged in firesetting; five, stolen without confrontation of a victim on more than one occasion; and six, stolen with confrontation of a victim.
>
> Then the next criteria [*sic*] is a pattern of irresponsible and antisocial behavior since the age of 15 as indicated by at least four of the following, and then they list another group.
>
> The four—actually I found one, two, three, four, five of the following: Unable to sustain a consistent work behavior, failure to conform with social norms with respect to lawful behavior as indicated by repeatedly performing antisocial or criminal acts, is irritable and aggressive as indicated by repeated physical fights or assaults, has no regard for the truth as indicated by repeated lying, and finally, is reckless regarding his own or others' personal safety as indicated by driving while intoxicated or recurrent speeding.
>
> Then the final category that he fits is that occurrence of antisocial behavior is not exclusively during the course of schizophrenia or manic episodes. He suffers from neither manic illness or schizophrenia so he fits all the criteria for antisocial personality disorder.[32]

While it hardly seemed necessary, given the evidence that Mr. Rouse had attended college, I also testified that in my opinion he was not mentally retarded. Based upon my interview with him, I had found Rouse to be of average or better intelligence.

The district attorney also used my testimony to explain the significance of Dr. Miller's admission that she approached the evaluation in this case as she would have approached any other case in her clinical practice. I tried to briefly explain, in a way the jury could understand, the distinction between a clinical and a forensic evaluation:

> If you are evaluating someone forensically, the first thing you have to be aware of is that there is this motivation to lie because generally when you are called in to do a forensic evaluation, the defendant's guilt or innocence or sometimes his sentence rides on what you have to say; and so the first thing you have to do is to be very, very concerned about getting the details, following up with a lot of questions and comparing everything the defendant tells you to every piece of evidence you can get from other sources and to be alert for inconsistencies.
>
> You don't do the same kind of evaluation in this kind of case that you would do if somebody just walked into your office and said, I'm having marital problems or trouble at home or trouble with my kids.[33]

Finally, on direct examination, I explained why Rouse did not meet the criteria for idiosyncratic alcohol intoxication:

> There are three criteria for that diagnosis. The first is maladaptive behavioral changes. That is aggressive or assaultive behavior that occurs within minutes of ingesting an amount of alcohol insufficient to produce intoxication in most people.
>
> The reason the defendant doesn't meet that criteria [*sic*] is because by his own statements he was drinking heavily, although he claims he was not intoxicated, he says he was drinking heavily that night. This [diagnosis] refers to an amount of alcohol insufficient to induce intoxication in most people.

> Second criterion is that the behavior is atypical of the person when not drinking, and here again, by his own statements to me and to the other doctors, this is a man with an explosive temper who frequently acts out in rages. So his behavior on the night in question was not atypical of his behavior generally.
>
> The final criteria [*sic*] is not due to any physical or other mental disorder. It's impossible to say whether or not he meets that criteria [*sic*]. He may, but two out of three he fails to meet.[34]

Cross-examination of an expert witness frequently focuses on what the expert failed to do, and this case was no exception. Michael Vavonese, Rouse's court-appointed defense attorney began cross-examination by chiding me for not having prepared a written report in this case:

Q: You still haven't given me a report; is that correct?

A: I have never prepared one.

Q: And you never—let me ask you this. Do you teach your law students to not have their psychologists prepare reports, Professor?

A: I think it's good to have a report if you can get one. You can't get one on a week's notice from a person as busy as me. . . . [A] report of the scope of Dr. Miller's which I think is the appropriate scope . . . would take hours and hours.[35]

I thought Vavonese's questions, though perhaps sarcastic, were fair, given that this was cross-examination. I also was not concerned about the questions because I felt I had a reasonable answer. The judge, however, was incensed by the defense attorney's questions and his tone. As soon as Vavonese finished this line of questioning, the judge sent the jury out and tore into the defense attorney:

> I must say that you were assigned to this case last August. You advised me at that time that you were going to use the insanity defense. . . .
>
> From what I am gathering, your doctor did not ever see [Rouse] until the 9th day of December. The district attorney had absolutely no way

> of knowing whether you were going to use that defense until you say, I have a doctor that will certify to this, he has no way of knowing whether the defense will be interposed.
>
> So as a practical matter, he has to wait until you get your report in. Now it has been testified to that that report came in the first part of January. . . . [I]t was your delay that caused this. Had you filed a report in October or November or December, the district attorney in my opinion would have an obligation to promptly answer that as best he could. . . . [F]or you now to badger this witness, who is a professional, is entitled to be treated with courtesy in this court, and I am going to demand it from here on out, over something that is ultimately your fault in my opinion is improper. . . . I really don't think it is proper for you to badger him over something that you know he had no control over. . . . If you want to attack him on his findings, if you want to attack him on his diagnosis, you do it; but you are attacking him on something he had nothing to do with, and that is filing a report. Your last statement was, don't you teach your students to file a report? Now, you know he didn't have time to file a report because you in fact were late. You are the one that caused that.[36]

Once we were past the issue of the report, I was surprised that there was almost nothing of any substance raised in the rest of the cross-examination. Instead, the defense attorney continued what I saw as a standard but probably not very useful indirect attack on my opinion. Vavonese pointed out, for example, that I was a psychologist and not a physician, I could not prescribe medications, I was being paid for my time, I would be paid by the District Attorney's Office, I had a law degree and was a law professor, I was "practiced in types of questions to ask witnesses,"[37] and I had not given the prosecutor my opinion until the day before I testified.

Perhaps the defense lawyer was simply laying the foundation for his attack on me during the closing arguments. In his closing to the jury, Vavonese compared Dr. Miller and me, both directly and indirectly:

> Now, let me tell you a few things about Dr. Miller. You know her credentials as a doctor, as a medical doctor, as a psychiatrist, and you were able to size her up when she testified. Listen, and I mean this in the

> most sincere way, she is a person of little style but of immense substance. She is not a professional witness. She is not a hired gun. She told you that she had only testified a few times before but she didn't have to tell you that. You could tell by the way she testified. You remember her insistence on reading from her notes. Sometimes I couldn't even kind of direct her. I couldn't control her; and her insistence on reading from the report, despite the fact that that is not always the way that it is done in a courtroom. . . . [W]hen the prosecution cross-examined her, and he cross-examined her cleverly, and he cross-examined her like a good, professional lawyer, what he tried to convince you was that there was something wrong in her taking time to prepare the report and that he went a bit too far when he did that. He tried to equate the fact that she took time to prepare her report with the fact that Dr. Miller wasn't being truthful, and that is just wrong. Say what you want about Dr. Miller but that is just wrong. . . .
>
> Dr. Miller didn't come in here as somebody who was handling complexities of the human situation and try to reduce that complex situation to simplistic answers. She didn't claim to have every answer. She came in here as a competent physician and as a decent and truthful human being and she told you what she believes because she believes it.
>
> We didn't hear from a medical doctor, from a psychiatrist, on the other side of this case. What the prosecution brought you was a lawyer with a psychology degree and what you heard from Dr. Miller was a physician giving her professional diagnosis. You heard from a person who works day in and day out with mental illness, who treats it, who empathisizes [*sic*] with it, who suffers with her patients, who feels with them. She is a doctor who came to testify, not a practiced witness with a psychology background.
>
> Maybe she lacks some of the suave and the charisma of the law professor who was clearly a trained witness but I will tell you one thing about Dr. Miller, I will tell you one thing about her, she understands mental illness.[38]

District Attorney Carbonaro felt the need to answer Vavonese's comparison only briefly. In the prosecution's closing, he told the jury:

> I submit to you, ladies and gentlemen, that Dr. Miller prepared a report, that she made some findings, that she found out she was wrong, that she

> had been lied to, and I submit to you that because of her credentials, she was afraid to back off of that opinion. That is what I submit, ladies and gentlemen.
>
> Dr. Ewing didn't have a written report prepared and turned over to defense counsel and we will grant you that and he conceded that; and I submit to you that there was good reason for that as well; and you know exactly what it was, that he didn't have an opportunity to examine this defendant until last Thursday, that there were certain documents that he wasn't provided with and had not an opportunity to review until just yesterday. For that reason, he held off preparing any report because he simply didn't have the time to do that and because if he did, he wouldn't have had all the facts that were available for him to review in front of him when he made up his mind and when he gave that decision.[39]

The last word to the jury regarding my testimony and that of Dr. Miller came from the judge. In fairly standard instructions, he told the jury:

> Now, there was some expert testimony in this case. Now, expert testimony is proper evidence to be considered by the jury and the law allows and permits an expert or person learned in a particular subject or field not only to testify to facts but also to give his opinion based upon such facts. This is allowed because an expert is supposed to, from his past experience, research and study, to have a peculiar knowledge upon the subject of the inquiry and an expert is supposed to be more capable than a layman in drawing conclusions from the facts and basing opinions upon them.
>
> Now, three experts who come to mind are Dr. Miller, Dr. Ewing and Dr. [Lazzaro]. . . .
>
> In determining the value of the testimony of any expert, whether he merely gives facts as to science or whether he gives facts and also some opinion testimony, you should consider his learning, his professional standing, his opportunity for study and his experience or her experience, his or her opportunity to observe the defendant, how they went about it, what they used and all such matters.
>
> The purpose of expert testimony is to aid you in your deliberations as to those matters upon which the expert is permitted to testify. Such testimony is merely a guide to you in your deliberations.

> Again, a jury at all times is the determiner of the facts. Expert testimony should not either be accepted or rejected indiscriminately. It should be weighed and considered by you the same as any other evidence.
>
> After weighing and considering such testimony, you are at liberty to disbelieve it when it is improbable or incredible or if you believe the expert witness has testified falsely or is mistaken.
>
> On the other hand, you are at liberty to accept it and act on it if you find that the testimony is based on underlying facts which have been established and the expert knew what he was talking about or she was talking about.
>
> The weight and value of an expert's testimony and his or her credibility is for you, the jury to decide. Put another way, as I said, an expert's testimony must be evaluated by you on the same tests that you would otherwise use and you must accept what you deem worthy of belief, reject what you don't deem worthy of belief and apply what weight you feel it deserves.[40]

After the judge completed his instructions, the jury deliberated for about two hours before finding Jimmy Lee Rouse guilty of murder, attempted murder, and unlawful use of an automobile. The following week, the judge dismissed the charge of unauthorized use of a motor vehicle and sentenced Rouse to the maximum prison terms for attempted murder and murder—12.5 years to life and 25 years to life, respectively—to be served consecutively, meaning that Rouse would not even be eligible for parole before serving 37.5 years behind bars. In sentencing Rouse, the judge told him, "Your record speaks loudly. You're a second violent felony offender," and then added, somewhat ironically, "It's obvious that you have no control over your emotions or actions. Like the psychiatrist said, you have a short fuse."[41]

CHAPTER 4

Insanity, Extreme Emotional Disturbance, or Both?

4

To the casual observer, John Justice was the perfect son. As a high school senior, he cleaned the meat department at a local supermarket from 8 PM to midnight but managed to earn top grades. A polite, quiet, and brilliant boy some regarded as a bit of a "nerd," John took care of his younger brother when his parents were working. Always eager to learn, he spent at least one day a week at the public library reading newspapers and news magazines, was worldly beyond his years and his small town, working-class circumstances, and had set his sights on attending a top university such as Harvard or Yale. With his honor grades and high SAT scores, attending an Ivy League school was a real possibility for John, who was accepted at two colleges during his junior year. His high school chemistry teacher called him "the kind of kid you loved to teach"[1] and added that "John ranks as one of the best students I have ever had."[2]

Much of what others saw in John was true. He was a devoted son, brother, employee, and student. But for years he had been depressed and obsessing daily over an incident that occurred when he was eight years old. On that occasion, John's mother had found John and a neighbor girl together naked and threatened to tell his father of the incident. Not long afterward, unknown to his family, John tried to kill himself.

In the years that followed, John was bullied at school. His peers pushed him around, beat him up, and poked fun at his clothing and footwear. Despite outward appearances, things were not any better for John at home. His father was often physically abusive to his mother and his younger brother, Mark. The police were frequently called to the Justice home to break up altercations between John's parents or to investigate neighbors' complaints about the behavior of his troubled brother.

While John's father did not abuse him physically, he certainly did so psychologically. In the presence of John's nuclear and extended family, his father frequently made references to John's lack of interest in athletics and girls. Frequently he called John a "faggot," "filthy kid," or any one of a number of other derogatory names.[3] The elder Justice made fun of his son's teenage acne, his broken eyeglasses that were held together by a piece of tape, and even the way he wore his hair, parted in the middle. He also mocked his son's interest in collecting models as a worthless hobby and laughed at John when he showed him his report cards.

By the time John reached high school, he had (unknown to his parents) twice tried to kill himself. By the age of 13, John was bigger than his father and felt that his size and presence sometimes deterred his father from beating his mother and brother. Still, John blamed himself for not intervening directly to protect them. Irrationally, he also blamed himself for his mother's demanding factory job, her failing health, his father's excessive drinking and abuse of the family, and his younger brother's apparently serious psychopathology. Not only did John blame himself for these problems, he traced all of them to the incident that occurred when he was eight years old, which had undoubtedly been long-forgotten by everyone except John.

Outside the home, John began to notice that his brother Mark, who was about five years younger, was becoming the kind of scapegoat and punching bag John had been for years. John felt that his brother was badly disturbed emotionally and that being bullied was making Mark's psychological problems worse. While John had been unable to protect himself from the bullies, he was now the size of a grown man, indeed bigger than many grown men, and didn't hesitate to step in to protect Mark from his tormentors.

High school brought John some respite as he threw himself wholeheartedly into his studies and became one of the top students in his class. Except for his grade in a typing class, John was a straight-A student. But even his academic achievements failed to put him in the mainstream of his peers. As one of his classmates said, "He wasn't a typical honors student. He really *hated* high school. If he got a poor grade on a test, he'd be so devastated that he'd be uncommunicative for a week. He put so much pressure on himself."[4]

Though John had but a single friend in high school and was still regarded by many as a nerd, he took comfort in all that he was learning—at school and on his own—and in the anticipation that before long he would leave home for college.

But those hopes were dashed when, as he completed his junior year of high school, his mother made it clear that the family could not help John financially with college and wanted him to stay at home and attend the local state university, where the education was good and tuition for in-state residents was quite inexpensive. John chafed at the idea of spending another four years with or near his troubled family and giving up his dream of attending a school commensurate with his intellect and talents. He worked as hard as he could at school and in his part-time job, but quickly realized that his dream of escaping was slowly but surely slipping away.

On Sunday, September 15, 1985, less than two weeks after the then 17-year-old had begun his final year of high school, John argued with his mother over a trivial matter—when he was going to do the dishes. John, who had to work that night and attend school the next day, was eager to leave the house and do some shopping before heading to his job. His mother forbade him to leave before he did the dishes and issued an ultimatum: John could do as he was told or move out and go live with relatives.

That night at the supermarket, John was unable to work and spent most of his time obsessing about his family. He was especially distraught to think that he could have done something so awful that his mother would tell him to leave home. As in the past, John blamed himself for his family's troubles. And while he had thought of it before, now an idea crystallized: he would put an end to the family's problems by killing them all and then committing suicide. By the end of his shift at midnight, he had no particular plan but had resolved to kill his family and himself.

John slept well that night, at peace with himself for the first time in years. By the time he arose from bed at 6:30 AM, he had the beginnings of a plan. He drove his father to work and agreed to pick him up at the end of his shift. That way, John could have the car for the day, a key element in his evolving homicidal plan.

When John returned from driving his father to work, he found himself alone in the house. Instead of heading to school, he called in sick and spent the morning and early afternoon alone cruising the town, at times driving as fast as 100 miles per hour in 30-mile speed zones.

After eating lunch at a fast-food restaurant, John returned home at about 1 PM, took two or three knives from his father's collection of hunting weapons, and began stabbing pillows and upholstered chairs before settling in front of the television to wait for his brother. When Mark came in from school, John followed him, struck him with a bat, stabbed him to death and then covered his body with a blanket.

John's mother was due home in half an hour. He sat and waited for her and, when she arrived, he stabbed her repeatedly in the back until she fell down a flight of stairs. Mortally wounded, Mrs. Justice asked John to call an ambulance. His only response was, "You're going."[5]

After killing his mother, John sat and thought for about 30 or 40 minutes until it was time to get his father. Before leaving to pick up Mr. Justice, John stopped to change his bloody pants so as not to arouse his father's suspicions. John drove the one or two miles to the plant where his father worked, explained that he was tired, and suggested that Mr. Justice drive the car home—so that John would be in a better position to kill his father when they arrived. Once Mr. Justice entered the home, John pulled a knife and stabbed him several times. As Mr. Justice lay dying, he asked "Where's Mary?"[6] John responded, "She's dead.

We're all dead."[7] John then stabbed himself in the arm, cut his wrist and his throat and waited to bleed to death. When it became apparent that he would not die from these self-inflicted wounds, John took some pills, which he soon vomited.

After drinking some liquor, John took a phone call from his uncle, who was looking for John's mother. John said she was out shopping, hung up the phone, and wrote a note. Feeling that the note made no sense, John burned it and, in doing so, set off a smoke detector. John dismantled the smoke detector and wrote another note: "I did this. This had to be done. This family should have had better. This was out of love not hate. John D. Justice."[8]

After completing the second note, which he left in the house, John immediately took off in the car, planning to crash the vehicle and kill himself. Driving roughly 90 miles per hour, John drove into a parked car that, unknown to John, was occupied by one of his neighbors, 22-year-old Wayne Haun. Though knocked unconscious, John suffered only minor injuries. Haun was killed in the crash.

When police officers and paramedics responded to the collision, John told them, "I killed my family." Seeing no one else with John in the car, one officer replied, "What do you mean? There's no one else here." To which John replied, "No, at home."[9]

After the officers read John his *Miranda* warnings, according to the police the following dialogue ensued:

John: "I'll answer your questions."

Officer: "What about your family?"

John: "Check 308 Mang. I killed them all."

Officer: "How?"

John: "With a kitchen knife."

Officer: "Who did you kill?"

John: "My father John W. Justice, my mother, Mary D. Justice, my brother Mark William Justice."

Officer: "When?"

John: "Last night."

Officer: "What were you doing since then?"

John: "I've been in the house. I tried to take pills but I couldn't swallow them."

Officer: "What happened with the accident?"

John: "I hit him on purpose. I wanted to kill myself."[10]

In an ambulance on his way to the hospital, John told paramedics, "I know I killed them. I had a reason. I'll remember it when I calm down."[11]

John was charged with three counts of intentional murder for the deaths of his mother, father and brother, and one count of "depraved indifference" murder in the death of Wayne Haun. Although John had no history of psychological or psychiatric treatment, it soon became evident that, at the very least, he had significant emotional problems. A county psychiatrist who examined him within two days of the killing found him suffering from an "acute psychosis."[12]

Since there was no question that John had committed the crimes charged, the only triable issue in the case was his state of mind at the time of the killings. Under New York's insanity defense statute, John could not be found criminally responsible if a jury found that, by reason of mental disease or defect, he lacked substantial capacity to know or appreciate either: (1) the nature and consequences of his conduct or (2) that his conduct was wrong when he killed his family and Wayne Haun.

John pleaded not guilty by reason of insanity and went to trial supported by the testimony of Dr. Emanual Tanay, a renowned Detroit psychiatrist who, at the time, was probably the leading authority on children who kill their parents. Tanay testified that based on his examination of John and review of the records in the case, John "suffers from a classic, chronic psychiatric illness."[13] "Specifically," Tanay explained, "I believe that that psychiatric illness most likely is schizophrenia."[14] The psychiatrist added that: "I say most likely because we are dealing still with a young individual. He's 17 years old, and schizophrenia develops in young adulthood and he doesn't show the classic picture of schizophrenia as yet. But it is my opinion that most likely the psychosis that he suffers from is schizophrenia."[15]

Asked by defense counsel, Joel Daniels, why John killed his family and tried to kill himself, Tanay replied, "Because he is and was psychotic. There is no other conceivable explanation."[16] Tanay went on to explain that, as a result of this psychosis, John "did not have the capacity to know or appreciate the nature and consequences of his conduct [and] did not have the capacity to know or appreciate that that conduct was wrong."[17] Asked about the diagnosis of a mere personality disorder given in a report by the prosecution's psychiatrist, Tanay said he disagreed: "[T]o say that someone who has engaged in this kind of behavior with even this kind of history, suffers from personality disorder would be as quote essentially normal, I find totally unacceptable."[18]

Tanay's direct testimony was smooth and concise, but he ran into trouble on cross-examination. Prosecutor Albert Ranni (now deceased) was a fiercely competitive litigator who had once been admonished by an appeals court for referring to a defendant's alibi witnesses and their testimony as "garbage" and "lies," and telling the jury that "We should wash that chair [the witness chair] after she [defendant's alibi witness] leaves."[19]

Ranni's cross-examination of Tanay had almost nothing to do with John Justice, his mental condition, or his crimes. The prosecutor spent nearly all his cross-examination attacking Tanay, and thus indirectly his opinion.

Although Tanay repeatedly pleaded that Ranni was taking his words out of context, the prosecutor skillfully used Tanay's own writings against him. For example, he forced Tanay to admit that he had once written that in most homicide cases in which the victim was in a close family relationship to the perpetrator, the perpetrator would qualify for an insanity defense. Tanay was also forced to acknowledge that in his view, such cases constituted about 60 to 80 percent of all homicides and that he believed that the insanity defense was underutilized in intrafamilial homicide cases. Ranni also pressed Tanay to acknowledge that he had written that most murderers are not criminals, but "decent, law-abiding, church-going" people.[20] Moreover, Ranni managed to force Tanay to agree that among 54 homicide cases he had evaluated, he had "found eighty-four percent of [the perpetrators] suffered from either dissociative reaction or schizophrenia."[21]

At times during the cross-examination, Ranni goaded Tanay into losing his professional demeanor. At one point, Tanay turned to the judge and said, "Your honor, he yells into my ear. I really think he is being argumentative. . . . I am referring to the court the fact that the prosecutor comes close to me, screams at me, and I find it really rude, number one. I am not some criminal accused of improper behavior. I don't think I should be treated that way."[22] The judge responded, "Thank you, Doctor. Mr. Ranni, utilize the podium. Go ahead."[23]

Still, Tanay managed to score a couple of points of his own on cross-examination, though neither had anything to do with John Justice. When Ranni got Tanay to acknowledge that most of his expert testimony was as a defense witness and that he had never reviewed a file for a prosecutor, Ranni made one of the biggest mistakes a cross-examiner can make, he asked the witness "Why?" Once a cross-examiner asks a witness "Why?" the witness has free rein to give a narrative answer and all the questioner can do is listen to the answer. Tanay, an experienced witness, seemed to sense this. He replied: "The reason is that it is well known that I will give an honest opinion. . . . And the prosecutor has to turn over that opinion to the defense lawyer. The prosecutors, generally, at least in my view, like to know ahead of time what the expert's opinion will be. With me you will not know ahead of time. You will only know after I examine."[24]

When Ranni implied that Tanay had formed his opinion in an earlier case and then looked to see if there were any discrepancies between what the defendant told him and what he told others, Tanay turned the tables on the prosecutor, replying, "Well, sir, I don't assume that the patient lied to me. Now, if you assume that he did, then please prove it to me. . . . I am not clairvoyant. It might turn out that it was inaccurate. If you have that information, please let me know."[25] The best Ranni could come back with was an unsubstantiated assertion that, in that particular case, the judge hearing the case convicted the defendant even though Tanay, testifying for the defense, was the only expert witness called by either side.

The real rebuttal of Tanay's opinion came from the testimony of Russell Barton, the prosecution's expert. Barton was a physician—indeed, like Tanay, a board-certified psychiatrist. While he held himself out to the public as an MD and was often referred to as "Dr. Barton" in court, he did not possess that degree or any other doctoral degree. Barton, who carefully avoided any mention of his degrees while testifying as to his qualifications in the Justice case, held an MBBS (Bachelor of Medicine and Bachelor of Surgery), a British undergraduate degree in medicine. He could have qualified for an MD degree in his native land had he conducted research and completed a doctoral thesis, but he never did so. Interestingly, under New York law, Barton could have qualified to use the title "MD" if he had bothered to register and pay a fee, but he had never done that either. In later cases in which Barton testified, his use of the MD degree would become a routine point of contention. In this trial, however, his educational background was apparently assumed to include that degree.

After relating the history John had given him as well as John's account of the killings, Barton testified that at the time of the crimes John was not suffering from schizophrenia, but rather from a personality disorder that "doesn't fit into any of the criteria for diagnosis inclusion in the *DSM-III*."[26] Barton explained that he reached this diagnosis in part because "[John] wasn't able to form friends. Perhaps he was too egocentric at times. He wasn't able to secure a girlfriend. He's never had a girlfriend although he was—"[27]

Ranni, apparently surprised by this explanation—or at least pretending to be—said, "I hope that is not evidence of a mental disorder, not having a girlfriend."[28] To which Barton gave a rather convoluted and cryptic, if not strange, reply:

> No, not in and of itself, no score does not make a game. But usually a young man of 18, 17, 18, the time comes when he becomes involved with some of those areas. But I think the defendant would feel he did

> not have enough time for girls and he couldn't see the human thing of it. I mean, that was a very stressing thought. And I think that we have been tied up with the feeling that this encounter has to be taken into consideration here. I think furthermore that he didn't have the kind of friends, and this again is an example of maladaptive, he had friends who would be described as nerds. These are school guys who are interested in intellectual pursuits and not too hung up with football and dances or other things which might be connected with your school background, and I think the fact that he was with this kind of interested and intellectual pursuit group, because he didn't have friends who might have been interwoven with the school background or who might have other direct pursuits than that of a Harvard-type school show that this again is maladaptive.[29]

Asked by Ranni whether "people sometimes commit bad acts even when they have that capacity to differentiate right and wrong,"[30] Barton gave another rambling and mystifying answer:

> Well, when we are talking about, when you say killing someone, then yes, of course, that would be. I mean, history is filled with barbarism. Minorities, horses coming down in full roar and they are trying to execute the whole gang, whether it was muscles or ammunition in '64, whether it is the Ku Klux Klan executing people or these terrible things. And I don't think that the average person, if they get into a situation where they commit a murder, obviously are committing, as we believe that, mutilation. We feel we could never wash our hands. I think this is very chivalrous but it is not lived out in history. It is barbarism where all the people get killed. Man is basically a vicious animal. He has binocular vision to seize his prey. He does not need an eye or shake his head. He had prehensile grip to seize his prey. I think we have to look at the people at this point that survived. There are many of us who develop a larger plan which controls and regulates these basic areas of passion. And the worst thing is so many people and regulations for those people are problems and the question arises because perhaps it at times gets out of control. And I decided to research this terrible thing, and suddenly mental illness from all his actions carried out in a sort of muddled way,

> in anger, in fury, I cannot firmly come up with this feeling. He felt they should have been done and he did them.[31]

Interestingly, Barton not only testified that John did not suffer from a mental illness but made it a point to add that even John did not believe that he suffered from any mental illness. John's claim that he suffered no mental illness, of course, could easily have been a symptom of his mental illness—many if not most schizophrenics lack insight into their mental illnesses. But John's stated belief that he was not mentally ill would also undercut the possibility that John was malingering mental illness since the malingerer wants the evaluator to believe that he is mentally ill.

Barton also testified that John not only knew what he was doing when he killed his family and neighbor but knew that the killings were wrong—that is, that John was not insane. To amplify and illustrate that conclusion, Ranni asked Barton if John would have committed these killings if there had been a uniformed police officer standing beside him at the time. This "policeman at the elbow" test of insanity, though often used by prosecutors to make a point, was clearly not a fair characterization of the New York insanity law described earlier. Barton's short answer was "No."[32] His explanation was longer:

> [John] decided that he would carry out the actions sequentially, that if he did it on Sunday, the whole family would be there and he wouldn't be able to reach his objective. So he decided to wait until Mark came in, get rid of him, which he regretted because he was quite fond of Mark. The reason he got rid of Mark, he told me, was, well, he might have run out of the home screaming or he might have called the police. So his own ideas, [if] the policeman had been there [he] could have interfered with the progression of his action, the completion of his plan and again he planned this so that he could do each individual piecemeal so they couldn't interfere with the second part of the plan, the killing of his mother, the third part, the collection and killing of his father. So I think that had the policemen been there, the restriction of his behavior would have been as I described, he wouldn't have done this.[33]

Barton was cross-examined by Joel Daniels, John's defense attorney, who had spent months preparing for this moment and came, as they say, loaded for bear. Like Ranni's cross-examination of Tanay, Daniels's cross of Barton was not about John Justice but rather about the witness.

Daniels's questioning began with a sequence that appeared to be about John Justice but was really an effort to challenge Barton's opinion that John was in no way mentally ill and to mock the British-born psychiatrist's rambling and often convoluted explanations of John's behavior, some of which were filled with dubious allusions to history:

Q: Doctor, is John Justice a member of the Stern gang?

A: I don't know. I shouldn't think so. Stern gang was back in the'50s [*sic*]. . . .

Q: Was he a member of the Ku Klux Klan?

A: I have no evidence that he was.

Q: Was he one of the Barbarians who descended on Rome?

A: No.

Q: Around ad 500?

A: No.

Q: Was he present when Lady Macbeth told her husband to commit the grievous and bizarre murders.

A: No, That was all fiction. I mean, we don't know that it really happened. . . .

Q: Tell me something, does the average teenager, red-blooded American boy stab his mother twelve times and push her down the cellar stairs because she uses $15 probably intended for a college application for a Buffalo Bills ticket?

A: No.

Q: Does the average red-blooded American boy, common everyday teenager stab his brother and father because the mother and father held hands together?

A: No.

Q: Does the average red-blooded American apple pie teenager stab his mother and his father and his brother because his parents might have had what is believed to be a love/hate relationship?

A: No.[34]

Next Daniels turned to another case in which Barton had testified that the defendant was neither mentally ill nor insane. In that case, the defendant, a young man with a history of mental problems had, for no apparent reason, killed his landlady. Daniels asked, "Well, anyway, he wanted to get rid of the devil because he thought the devil was inside the building and he chopped her head off and stabbed her over thirty times, isn't that right?"[35] To which Barton replied, "No. He chopped off her head because she wouldn't jump out of the window."[36]

Daniels then turned to a standing contract Barton had with the district attorney's office in a nearby county, under which Barton was paid to give testimony for that prosecutor's office. The defense attorney and expert witness quarreled over the meaning of the contract, Daniels implying that it showed Barton was basically on the DA's payroll and routinely did their bidding, and Barton claiming that the highly unusual written agreement was nothing more than a form of bookkeeping that allowed him to be paid for his services.

But Daniels was not about to let Barton wiggle off the hook so easily. He got Barton to acknowledge that in the 40 to 50 times he had testified, he had "always come into court at the request of the District Attorney and found the defendant to be legally sane."[37] He also forced Barton to admit that in one such case, in the county in which he was under contract with the DA's office, he had been summoned to a local police station by an assistant district attorney from the office to examine an arrested murder suspect on the spot. Knowing that the man,

James Riley, had not yet spoken to a lawyer, Barton conducted a one-hour psychiatric interview to determine whether he was insane. Riley, who had killed his wife and three children, pleaded insanity, and was convicted of murder after Barton later testified at trial that he suffered only a personality disorder and was not insane.

Daniels asked Barton, "Doctor, was seeing this defendant before he had a lawyer to determine his psychiatric status a violation of ethical standards of the American Psychiatric Association?"[38] Daniels was referring to that aspect of the American Psychiatric Association's Code of Ethics which read: "Ethical considerations in medical practice preclude the psychiatric evaluation of any person charged with criminal acts prior to access to, or availability of, legal counsel. The only exception is the rendering of care to the person for the sole purpose of medical treatment."[39]

Initially Barton replied "That I don't know."[40] Daniels then produced the transcript of Riley's trial, in which Barton had been asked on cross-examination about the ethics of his conduct in the case. Barton then testified "I don't know at what time that [the ethical standard in question] came in, that's recent, the formulation of the so-called ethical rules is more recent, but I am not sure."[41] Asked if he had ever read the code of ethics, Barton replied, apparently as if to minimize their importance to psychiatric practice and/or to explain his stated ignorance of the code, "Don't read all the numerous advertisements and reports, no."[42] Pressed relentlessly by Daniels, Barton finally grudgingly gave the answers the defense attorney seemed to be seeking:

Q: Were you familiar with the ethical consequences of seeing the defendant in the situation in which Mr. Riley found himself on January 7, 1985, prior to the time he had counsel, were you aware of that?

A: To the degree of awareness, yes, of course.

Q: Just like in this case, you are totally aware.

A: Totally aware.

Q: Isn't that right?

A: Yes, but then, of course, I know that this was, well, a matter which had been discussed and it has been discussed for many years.

Q: Yes.

A: I didn't know they actually formulated the written opinion at that time. I don't know who the committee was, but I know that my ethical standards are that I would not help to cheat a man who had not seen an attorney.

Q: You knew he had not seen a lawyer?

A: I knew he hadn't seen a lawyer, yes.

Q: Then you were cheating him, weren't you?

A: No, because I wasn't asking him about the facts. I was asking him about his mental state. I wasn't asking him whether he had done this or not.[43]

Next Daniels turned to Barton's credentials, requiring him to acknowledge that he was not board certified in forensic psychiatry. Barton testified that he did not approve of such certification. It was not clear that he appreciated the irony of his testimony that "I think psychiatrists should stick to psychiatry and not come to court."[44] Daniels asked, "So psychiatrists should not enter the courtroom?"[45] Barton replied, "Not at all, I don't think so, with their superficial knowledge of the law. They should stick with attending patients and so forth, not necessarily assisting but maybe in unique cases, and I think there are those, when it comes to court, it doesn't give them specialization with patients. It doesn't necessarily enable them to be impartial in part, you see."[46]

Barton's responses to this line of questioning were especially ironic in view of the testimony Daniels elicited from Barton shortly thereafter. Daniels confronted Barton with a copy of a letter the psychiatrist had written years earlier to the chairman of the Department of Psychiatry at a local medical school. In the letter, Barton had asked for a promotion to full professor from his position of clinical associate professor. In the letter, Barton noted that the requested promotion "has implications which could be or become important when giving evidence in court."[47] Daniels also forced Barton to acknowledge that he had never received even a response to the letter, much less any promotion.

Daniels's last major line of attack on Barton was one he had been preparing for months. He had learned that Barton had left England about a decade earlier under unpleasant circumstances precipitated by a *London Times* editorial criticizing Barton for an article he had published in 1968 regarding the Bergen-Belsen Nazi concentration camp, where it is generally recognized that members of the Third Reich killed or deliberately starved to death many thousands of Jews. According to Barton's own testimony the *Times* had written that he had described this concentration camp as "not too bad."[48]

In court, Daniels asked Barton flat out, "Did you say that the Nazi death camps weren't too bad?"[49] To which, Barton replied, "I quoted, that was in a statement that is in [my book] *Institutional Neurosis*."[50] After an objection by the prosecutor, Daniels repeated the question and the following colloquy ensued:

A: Well, I didn't say that. I quoted it.

Q: Did you say that—that the death camp conditions in many of the Nazi extermination camps were like mental hospitals in the United Kingdom and United States?

A: I attempted to draw the parallel, yes.

Q: You drew the parallel, did you?

A: Yes. . . .

Q: At the end of the war, did you go to the Bergen-Belsen concentration camp?

A: At the end of the war, the war was about over when I went there, yes.

Q: Did you spend a month there?

A: Yes, about . . .

Q: Over one hundred fifteen thousand people, mostly Jews, were killed there?

A: No, I don't think it was that number. The number was thirty thousand.

Q: You disagree with the statement that over one hundred fifteen thousand people, mostly Jews, were killed at Belsen.

A: Well—

Q: You disagree with it or do you agree with it?

A: I disagree with it. . . . It is very difficult to get reasonably reliable evidence as to what went on. There was brutality in Belsen, there is no question, but it wasn't widespread. It wasn't an extermination camp as opposed to Auschwitz and Buchenwald. . . .

Q: It was a very controversial article that you wrote, wasn't it?

A: Yes, it was.

Q: Did you leave England because of this article?

A: No.

Q: Did you also claim in this article I became convinced contrary to popular opinion there had never been a deliberate policy of starvation?

A: Yes.

Q: In other words, you claim that the Nazis and the SS did not deliberately starve to death men, women or children in Belsen?

A: Yes.

Q: That is not what inmates said, is it?

A: Not all of them. . . .

Q: They were starved to death, weren't they?

A: Some were quite plump.

Q: That a fact?

A: Yes. That surprised me, too.[51]

By this point in the trial, it may have appeared to the jury that Russell Barton was on trial, and in a sense he was. Daniels was trying hard to convince the jury that they should not give credence to the opinion of a physician who arguably had a clear bias against defendants, may have acted unethically in at least one earlier case, and may have discounted or at least minimized the Nazi atrocities of World War II.

Perhaps the only way to gauge Daniels's success in that regard is to look at the jury's verdict. The jurors could offer no direct verdict on Russell Barton, MBBS, but they did reach one on John Justice. And a rather strange one it was. Although all four of the killings had taken place during a roughly five-hour time period, the jury concluded that John was guilty of the intentional murder of his mother and the depraved indifference murder of Wayne Haun, but not guilty by reason of insanity in the killings of his brother and father. Taken at face value, that would mean that the jury concluded that John was insane when he stabbed his brother, then sane half an hour later when he killed his mother, and then insane again within an hour when he took his father's life, and that, somehow, after all three killings, a couple of hours later he was again sane when he drove into Wayne Haun's car and killed him.

Such a verdict defied not only logic but the testimony of both experts, Barton and Tanay. As it turned out, the jury had actually been torn between conviction and an insanity acquittal on all charges and had, in the end, reached this bizarre compromise.

Since John had been both convicted and acquitted by reason of insanity, it was initially unclear what would happen to him. Ultimately the court sentenced him to 25 years to life in prison and decided that he would be imprisoned rather than hospitalized. John went to prison and was treated for his mental illness as an inmate rather than a patient.

Over the next five years or so, he would be examined and treated by a dozen psychologists and psychiatrists, every one of whom diagnosed him as suffering from schizophrenia. During that period of time, John was treated with powerful antipsychotic medications and was in and out of prison psychiatric units.

In December 1991, five years after his combination conviction-acquittal, a state appellate court found that the verdicts were not inconsistent as a matter of law but reversed the murder convictions, explaining:

> The case should be sent back for a new trial, however, because the court's charge was inadequate, confusing and misleading. All the examples the court used in its original charge and supplemental charge to illustrate application of the insanity defense involved an individual who suffered from delusions or hallucinations. However, both Dr. Tanay, defendant's expert, and Dr. Barton, the People's expert, acknowledged that defendant did not suffer from delusions or hallucinations. Therefore, the jury could have been misled to believe that defendant was not insane solely for that reason.
>
> Moreover, the court failed to respond meaningfully to the jury's request for further instructions. The jury asked "can defendant be mentally ill and still be criminally responsible?" The court responded "[t]he answer to that question is yes." Answering the question with a simple "yes," without further explanation of the elements of the affirmative defense, did nothing to alleviate the jury's confusion and instead added to it, because the next question the jury asked was whether they could find defendant "guilty" by reason of insanity. The court, again, did not explain the elements of the affirmative defense and told the jury only that there were three possible verdicts as to each count—guilty, not guilty, or not responsible because of mental disease or defect.[52]

In his second trial, John would be represented by John Nuchereno, the attorney who had convinced the appeals court to grant a new trial. The case would be prosecuted not by Ranni but by another assistant district attorney, George Quinlan. Quinlan began the pretrial proceedings by telling the judge, that he "would let Justice plead guilty to second degree murder to settle the matter."[53] Nuchereno was unimpressed with this "offer." Had John taken the so-called offer and pleaded guilty to murder, the entire appeals process would have been for naught. Quinlan, an experienced prosecutor had to have understood that and could hardly have been surprised when Nuchereno told the court that a guilty plea to murder was "out of the question."[54]

Having researched juvenile homicide for years and having written two books on the subject, I was not surprised when Nuchereno called and asked me to examine John Justice. Before I did so, I met with Nuchereno who was the most well-prepared litigator I had ever met. He had already reviewed and mastered thousands of pages of records from John's first trial and his subsequent incarceration and mental health care. He asked me to do the same before I saw John and to take as long as I needed to do a thorough evaluation. As it turned out, that took well over 100 hours. In addition to reviewing the file and interviewing others, I spent a total of 25 hours examining John Justice on 14 separate occasions.

Having reviewed the records and thoroughly examined John, I reached the conclusion that he did, in fact, suffer from schizophrenia and that he was, at the time of the crimes, legally insane. The second trial shaped up—much as the first had—as a "battle of the experts." This time, some things would be the same and some would be different. Among the differences were the substitution of me for Tanay, and the backing of 12 other doctors who had examined John since his conviction six years earlier and unanimously diagnosed and treated him as schizophrenic. The one major similarity between the two trials was the identity of the state's expert. Having read the transcript from the first trial, I was initially quite surprised to learn that the prosecution planned to call Russell Barton as its only expert. The more I thought about it, however, the more that choice made sense, despite what had come out about Barton in the first trial. I and a dozen other doctors had examined John and found him suffering from schizophrenia. The only psychiatrist or psychologist who had examined John and disagreed was Barton, who testified in the first trial that John suffered from only a personality disorder and was poised to testify in the second trial that John was malingering—that is, pretending to suffer from symptoms of schizophrenia. Perhaps, I thought, Quinlan planed to present Barton again because Barton was all he had—the only expert he knew for sure would conclude that John was not schizophrenic.

John's second trial was also different in that this time his plea was not only insanity but extreme emotional disturbance. The acquittals for the killings of his father and brother were off the table; they could not be retried because John had been found not guilty, albeit by reason of insanity. All that were left to try the second time around were the deaths of John's mother and neighbor. The jury would have three possible verdicts in each of the two killings: guilty of murder, not guilty by reason of insanity, and guilty of manslaughter. If the jury concluded that, at the time of the killings, John was sane but acting in a state of extreme emotional disturbance for which there was a reasonable cause or explanation, they would be obliged to find him guilty of the lesser crime of manslaughter rather than murder.

In my direct testimony I explained to the jury my opinion that John suffered from schizophrenia and, as a result, was, when he committed the homicides, substantially unable to appreciate the nature and consequences and wrongfulness of his acts. I also explained my opinion that John was, as a result of this illness, in a state of extreme emotional disturbance at the time he killed his family and his neighbor.

On cross-examination, Quinlan did pretty much what I had anticipated he would, although there were a few surprises. I had been cross-examined by so many of Quinlan's colleagues in the Erie County District Attorney's Office that I knew their playbook well. Thus, I was not surprised when Quinlan re-established that I was not a medical doctor but a PhD and could not perform surgery, prescribe medications or order medical tests; I would be paid for my work on this case; I had never before testified on behalf of his employer, the Erie County District Attorney's Office; I, as a tenured full professor in a major university (in his words) "taught school"; I had previously testified on behalf of Judith Neelley, a convicted killer and death row inmate in Alabama; I had once given a lecture entitled "Ten Commandments for the Expert Witness," which was taped and sold commercially by a publisher, and not a single one of my commandments was to tell the truth; I had once appeared on a prime-time TV special, "Live from Death Row," hosted by Geraldo Rivera; I had an undergraduate degree in psychology that was a BA so psychology was one of the arts or at least not an "exact science"; and I had many years earlier been demoted by an employer for refusing to stop attempting to organize a labor union. Quinlan also asked me the apparently obligatory line of questions aimed at establishing that mental illness, per se, even one as serious as schizophrenia, does not necessarily equate to insanity as the law defines that term.

All of that I expected. What surprised were several lines of questioning that seemed either to serve no purpose or to serve one that benefited the defense. One had to do with a statement I made on direct examination. Quinlan pressed me on this point for no reason I can imagine, other then perhaps to play "who knows more about the Bible?" or to prolong the cross-examination, which lasted three or four days:

Q: Okay. So you're saying that mental disease at least in your opinion has been around since the time of Abel and Cain?

A: Well, it's a metaphorical statement. I don't know if I meant it absolutely, I didn't know Abel and Cain personally, but what I'm saying is from the—throughout the history of humankind, mental illness has been around.

Q: Well, are you familiar with the story of Cain and Abel?

A: Sure.

Q: As indicated in the scripture?

A: Yes.

Q: And actually Cain was found to have slain his brother Abel?

A: Right.

Q: And he was confronted by the Lord at that time, and was accused of having done just that, killing his brother Abel?

A: Right.

Q: Is that your understanding?

A: Pretty much.

Q: And as a matter of fact, the Lord, according to Book 4 of Genesis, asks Cain, what hast thou done, the voice of thy brother's blood crieth unto me from the ground. . . .

A: And the Lord said unto Cain, why art thou wroth and why is thy countenance fallen?

Q: Verse 11.

A: I got it.

Q: Now thou art cursed from the earth, which had opened her mouth to receive thy brother's blood from thy hand?

A: Right.

Q: And going on to verse 15, and the Lord said unto him therefore, whosoever slayeth Cain, vengeance shall be taken on him sevenfold, in other words, he says vengeance is mine, in regards to Cain?

A: The Lord.

Q: And the Lord set a mark upon Cain, lest any finding him should kill him. And that to this day has been known as the mark of Cain, and that's been the origin of the term, a marked man, true?

A: I guess.

Q: And yet you want to remove that mark that the court put on Cain and replace it with the mark of mental illness?

A: No.

Q: Okay. There was certainly no psychiatric defense at the time of Cain and Abel, was there?

A: No.[55]

In another exchange, Quinlan opened a door for the jury to hear what they otherwise would not have regarding the consequences of a finding of insanity. In New York, jurors are generally told only at the end of an insanity trial that if they find the defendant insane, further proceedings will be held. In other words, jurors are never told by the court that a defendant acquitted by reason of insanity will almost assuredly be indefinitely locked up in a state institution. In this case, the prosecutor tried to falsely paint me as believing that John should not be held accountable for the killings. As a result, he became angry with me, lost control of the cross-examination and watched his strategy backfire badly:

Q: Now, I have to go back to this for just a minute. Your—your opinion in this case, namely that the defendant should not be held accountable—

A: That's not my opinion.

Q: Well, your opinion is that his capacity to know and appreciate the nature and consequences of his act or that his act—or that his conduct was wrong is substantially impaired by a mental illness?

A: That's true.

Q: Therefore, he should not be held accountable.

A: Well, you—you and I both know that he'll be held accountable no matter what happens.

Q: Well—

A: The law doesn't speak in accountability, The—

Q: Well—

A: The law speaks in terms of responsibility.

Q: Well the defense here goes to whether or not he's going to be convicted of murdering his mother and Wayne Haun, true?

A: Yeah. Whether he goes to a state hospital for the criminally insane or to a mental institution.

Q: Well, you know darn well he's not going to go to a hospital, don't you?

A: If he's found not responsible?

Q: You know that that's the case, because you're testifying day in and day out in this courthouse to get these people out on the street, aren't you?

A: If he's found not responsible he's going back to a state prison for the criminally insane.

Q: Yes or no? Yes or no? And somebody like you is going to come along and suggest he should be out on the street, true?

A: I don't think he'll ever be out on the street.[56]

Defense attorney Nuchereno objected to Quinlan's statement "Well, you know darn well he's not going to go to a hospital." As Nuchereno argued,

> [I]t's not correct, and it's not the law in New York State.... [T]he instruction that the court has to give is that it's not a matter for the jury to worry about, but hearings will be held and involuntary confinement when appropriate, etcetera. Well, Mr. Quinlan has now planted the seed by making a statement ["]well, you know darn well he won't go to a hospital.["] This witness does not know darn well that that would take place. This witness does not know what would take place if there's a not responsible verdict, other than the fact that two psychologists or psychiatrists will examine the defendant and—and to determine whether he is ill and dangerous. And as an aside, I say that that's a foregone conclusion that they will determine that, but that's not relevant for what I'm stating here. So this jury now has the belief from an Assistant District Attorney that ["]well, you know darn well he won't go to a hospital.["] Now, judge, they've heard that.... This is going to be on their mind, and this is a most serious matter, and I think that would deprive my client of a fair trial. And I must ask for the strongest cautionary instruction that that isn't so.... I'm asking this court to do more than what the standard instruction is. It has to be put to them in the strongest possible terms that

> that's not true, the Assistant District Attorney was out of line to have said it, and it doesn't apply in this case, and they should disregard all that and strike that exchange.[57]

Though Quinlan blamed me for his inappropriate statement, telling the judge that it was triggered by my "gratuitous" and "nonresponsive" statement that preceded it, he offered to join Nuchereno's motion for a special instruction to the jury but requested that my statement be stricken as well.[58]

After a five-minute recess, the judge informed Quinlan that "I've reviewed that testimony to which we referred in our argument previously, and Mr. Quinlan, I cannot, I will not grant your request. I believe that the answer was responsive insofar as your question was concerned, and I will not grant your request."[59] Once the jury returned to the courtroom, the judge added the following statement:

> I want to give you the following information. Near the end of this morning's session when Mr. Quinlan was cross-examining Dr. Ewing, Mr. Quinlan made certain suggestions about the defendant not going to a hospital if he was found not responsible by reason of mental disease or defect. That line of questioning was totally improper, and Mr. Quinlan—Mr. Quinlan should not have asked those questions. The law provides . . . as follows: Where a defendant has raised the affirmative defense of lack of criminal responsibility by reason of mental disease or defect . . . the court must without elaboration instruct the jury as follows, and I instruct you in the following manner: A jury during its deliberations must never consider or speculate concerning matters relating to the consequences of its verdict. However, because of the lack of common knowledge regarding the consequences of a verdict of not responsible by reason of mental disease or defect I charge you that if this verdict is rendered by you there will be hearings as to the defendant's present mental condition, and where appropriate, involuntary commitment proceedings. So, as you can see, a verdict of not responsible by reason of mental disease or defect does not mean that someone is allowed to leave the courthouse free of any further proceedings. Therefore I have stricken Mr. Quinlan's line of questioning which suggests otherwise, and you

are—and you are to disregard it entirely. And his suggestions which were improper are to play no part at all in your ultimate consideration of this case.

And Mr. Quinlan, you are not to ask any questions like that in the future. Go ahead.[60]

Russell Barton was called to rebut my testimony. Again the psychiatrist denied that John was mentally ill or insane, but this time he had to go up against not just the opinion of one opposing doctor but the opinions of 13, all of whom had diagnosed John as schizophrenic *after* he had been convicted and sent to prison, and 12 of whom were state prison and mental health employees with not even an arguable ax to grind.

Barton's explanation? John was malingering, faking mental illness, he told the jury, and had fooled all 13 of us but could not fool him. What Barton could not explain, however, was why this young man, convicted of murder at the age of 18 and sentenced to 25 years to life in prison, would want to pretend for over five years that he was mentally ill, knowing that the consequence was that he would be prescribed powerful antipsychotic medications and subject to the probability of civil confinement in the event he was ever paroled. Nor could Barton explain why, if John were malingering, he denied having any mental illness, or why, at the end of his own examination of the defendant, John threw his hands up and told Barton "Look, I don't know why you're going through all this. They just spent six, seven years trying to convince me I'm mentally ill. I don't want to do this any more."[61]

Who did the jury believe? Barton? Me and my dozen concurring colleagues? Or none of us? We'll never know. But what we do know is that the jury acquitted John of murder, found that he had been suffering from an extreme emotional disturbance at the time of the two killings, and convicted him of the lesser crime of manslaughter. As a result of this verdict, John's life sentence was vacated and the question was no longer *if* he would ever be released from prison but *when.*

The judge answered that question when he sentenced John to the maximum prison term possible: thirteen and a third to 40 years. Under New York law, since John was incarcerated from the day of the killing and had already served over six and a one-third years behind bars, this sentence meant that he would be eligible for parole in seven years and that, with time off for good behavior, he would have to be conditionally released on parole in less than 14 years—that is, after he had served a total of 20 years.

In September 2005, John was released from prison. He had not taken any medications in years, had completed an associate's degree from Syracuse University while incarcerated, and was hoping to resume his education. Though John pleaded not to be returned to Buffalo, where his name and face were well known from the publicity surrounding his trials, parole authorities insisted that John enter a halfway house in Buffalo and that he accept outpatient treatment at the local state psychiatric center.

In the private-sector halfway house, which was run by an ex-convict, John was required to live with various criminals, including drug offenders, child molesters, robbers, and murderers. Initially John adjusted well to the halfway house and was accepted for admission to the local campus of the state university. But he was never satisfied with living at the halfway house, where he said he was exposed to drugs, guns, and various criminal activities and claimed he was pressured to participate in Christian religious activities.

After living there almost a year, John felt he was ready to move into an apartment of his own. Evidently parole authorities agreed but mental health officials, who still had authority over John under the two earlier insanity acquittals, refused to allow him to move. In what he described as a calculated decision aimed at being returned to prison, which he found preferable to the halfway house, John told the director of the halfway house that if he was not allowed to leave soon he might harm someone. The director contacted John's parole officer and John was soon returned to prison, where he again awaits parole.

Was John Justice schizophrenic, as I and a dozen other psychologists and psychiatrists concluded? Or was he malingering, as Russell Barton claimed? Neither I nor any other mental health professional except Barton has ever claimed to have seen any evidence that John was faking mental illness; indeed, while John acknowledged that he had been at times seriously depressed, he always adamantly maintained—and maintains to this day—that he has never been mentally ill.

When John was released from prison to the halfway house in 2005, I was appointed by the court to examine him to determine whether he was dangerously mentally ill. I saw none of the symptoms of schizophrenia I had seen when I examined him back in 1991, indeed I saw no symptoms of mental illness at all.

Schizophrenia is a lifelong illness, for which there is no cure. Schizophrenics sometimes have periods of remission wherein they show few if any symptoms of the illness, but long-term remissions are rare, especially when the patient is not taking any medications.

John may be one of those rare individuals who suffers from schizophrenia but is able to maintain a lengthy, even permanent remission. I hope that is the case. Better yet, though it would call into question the diagnostic accuracy of 13 psychologists and psychiatrists, including me, I hope that we were all wrong and that, despite his very real symptoms of mental illness in his teens and early 20s, John never suffered from schizophrenia.

CHAPTER 5

Voluntary or Coerced Confession?

5

When I was a first-year graduate student at Cornell University, I had a hard time finding an affordable place to live. Getting by on a small fellowship stipend left me living in a first-floor storefront that had been converted into an apartment of sorts on one of the main streets of Ithaca's "Collegetown." Not infrequently, people passing by would walk through my door without knocking, mistaking it for the entrance to a retail store. Each night, after I'd turned out the lights and gone to bed, I could hear the passing foot patrolman trying the door to make sure it was locked. I got a kick out of the people walking in, asking what was for sale, and found the police officer's nightly routine reassuring.

Though the accommodations were modest, to put it mildly, I felt entirely safe and comfortable until one night when I heard a commotion in the street. Stepping outside my door, I could see an ambulance and a slew of police officers. A man had been stabbed to death just a few feet from my Eddy Street apartment, the first homicide in the Ithaca area in several decades. For weeks afterward, the white outline of the body remained on the sidewalk, a silent testament that even this idyllic college community was not immune from the most violent of crimes.

Though I rarely thought of that murder once the body silhouette was finally washed away, the next school year I moved from Eddy Street into the countryside on the outskirts of Ithaca. There I rented the entire second floor of a small, two-family house for about what I had paid for my storefront apartment in Collegetown. Homes were spread out, the population was sparse, and I rarely saw anyone except at the nearby general store where I went daily to pick up my mail and purchase a TV dinner. I could not imagine a crime, much less a murder, taking place in that tranquil environment.

I left that apartment after my second year at Cornell and really never gave it much thought until many years later when I read in the *Buffalo News* about a brutal mass murder that took place just a proverbial stone's throw down the road from where I had once lived. In the most shocking, if the not worst, crime ever to hit the Ithaca area, Warren and Delores Harris and their two children were shot to death in their rural home on December 23, 1989. One of the children, a teenage girl, was brutally raped and sodomized before her death, and the unknown perpetrator had fled after trying to set the home on fire.

Though I had not lived in Ithaca for about 14 years and had been back for visits only rarely, I could well imagine the shock, grief, and outrage of the small community I had briefly called home. Crimes like the Harris killings just did not happen on the hill "high above Cayuga's waters" in the shadows of Cornell University. Drug deals, burglaries, a robbery every so often, and the occasional rape perhaps, but not murder, and certainly not murder as ugly as this one.

As I would later learn, the police had a difficult time solving this crime, and as the weeks went by, the pressure for an arrest mounted exponentially. Not only were town folks shocked, outraged, and fearful, they were angry at the police for not immediately arresting the culprit. If this could happen to the Harrises, a well-liked and affluent family with an expensive and elaborate alarm system, Ithacans reasoned, it could happen to anyone. Though the killer could simply have been passing through the area, no one seemed to believe that. Fueled in part by media speculation, the general consensus was that a vicious killer remained on the loose in Ithaca and that, until he was captured, no one was safe.

After days of apparently fruitless investigation, the police began to get a few breaks. Credit cards had been taken from the Harris home and used at an automatic teller machine and in several stores in a nearby mall. Store clerks were questioned without much success, but a local man and his son came forward to say that they had seen an African American couple at an ATM the day after the Harrises were killed. They remembered the couple, they told police, because the man was having trouble with the ATM, which he said had taken his card and would not give it back. As it turned out, the card "eaten" by the machine belonged to the Harrises. The man and his son gave descriptions of the couple to a forensic artist who created sketches of the duo.

The sketches were published in the local newspaper and several weeks later resulted in another break for the investigators. Nearly a month after the crime, a young woman told police that the female in one of the sketches resembled her coworker, Shirley Kinge. The male in the sketch, she said, looked like Shirley's son, Michael Kinge.

From there on, the investigation was easy, or so it seemed. Police quickly learned that 35-year-old Michael Kinge had a criminal record—including robbery, fraud, and use of a firearm with a silencer—and had served time in state prison. His mother Shirley, they learned, was 55 years old, had no criminal record, and shared a duplex with her son just outside Ithaca. Shirley shared her half of the house with her elderly mother, while Michael lived in the other half with his girlfriend and their infant son.

Once the Kinges were identified as suspects, police put them under round-the-clock surveillance, tracking their every move. Investigators obtained samples of Shirley's handwriting from her employer, and an expert reported that "in all probability" Shirley had signed the charge slips when the Harris's credit cards were used the day after the killings.[1]

Police had a mug shot of Michael as well as his fingerprints but no photograph or fingerprints of Shirley. To fill that gap in the investigation, David Harding, a state police officer went undercover, showed up as a guest at the bed and breakfast where Shirley worked, and did his best to get Shirley's picture, prints and more examples of her handwriting. Posing as a grant administrator visiting Cornell, Harding feigned a hand injury and talked Shirley into handing him a glass and helping him address some envelopes. Though he later retrieved the glass, Harding reported finding no usable prints. His effort to get Shirley's photograph, he said, was thwarted by her modesty.

Harding persisted, however, and eventually, on the pretext that he could help Shirley obtain a federal grant, tricked her into providing her Social Security number, date and place of birth, the names and addresses of her family members, her employment history, and all the places she had lived.

Armed with these data, Harding tracked down Shirley's work records. Since she had once worked for a government agency, her fingerprints were on file and were quickly turned over to Harding. Harding compared Shirley's prints to those found on a gas can at the scene of the murders and pronounced them a match.

While the undercover operation and surveillance of Shirley was fruitful, police had much less luck in the pursuit of evidence against Michael Kinge. Store clerks had been shown his mug shot and positively identified him as having used the Harris's credit cards. They still lacked evidence that would place Michael at the scene of the murders, but the store identifications, coupled with Michael's record and the evidence against his mother, convinced police that he had killed the Harris family. Shirley, they believed, may have been involved in the killings but, at the very least, was implicated in the arson that followed.

While the investigation and surveillance proceeded, Michael Kinge became well aware that he was a suspect in the Harris killings. Not only did the police question both him and his girlfriend, but they later tried to lure him out of his home by having a former employer call him with a bogus job offer, a ruse he quickly saw through. Meanwhile, one of Michael's acquaintances called and told Michael that the police had been asking about him. As the police became more and more convinced that Michael was their man, Michael became a recluse, refusing to leave his apartment for any reason.

On February 7, 1990, roughly seven weeks after the Harrises were killed, a team of seven New York State police officers stormed Michael' Kinge's apartment at dawn. According to the police accounts of the incident, Michael's back was turned to the officers; he had a shotgun and appeared poised to kill himself. "Don't do it, don't do it, don't do it," one officer reportedly yelled.[2] Another said he told Michael, "It's all over. Just give me the gun and things will be okay."[3] As that officer reached for the gun, Michael allegedly turned and fired the weapon. Immediately, the officers unleashed a volley of gunfire. Within seconds, nine shots were fired, and Michael Kinge was dead.

While all of this was happening, a second team of seven officers was forcing its way into Shirley's apartment on the other side of the duplex, where they knew they would find Shirley, her elderly mother, and Michael's infant son. Three police officers confronted Shirley, arrested her, and whisked her off to a state police barracks for questioning. Within a few hours, Shirley admitted that on the day after the Harris murders, Michael had come to her apartment and convinced her to go Christmas shopping with him. She recounted the fateful stop at the ATM and how the machine retained his card and explained that she did not understand why Michael had been so upset. In response to her questions, she said that he told her, "It's got my prints on it and if they find it I'm in trouble."[4]

As for the shopping trip to the mall, Shirley explained, "Michael said 'why don't you go and buy yourself something.' I told him that I didn't have any money. He reached into his pocket and he came out with this envelope and took a card out of the envelope and gave the card to me. He told me to use the card, saying that it was blank. He said that all I had to do was sign it and that I could use it. I asked him where he got it from and he said that he got it from a guy down by the Commons. He gave me the telephone number and address for me to use for identification."[5]

Asked for the name, address, and number, Shirley replied, "Delores E. Harris. I don't remember the phone number. It was 539-something. The address was 1885 Ellis Hollow Road, Ithaca, New York."[6] Asked what she did with the card, Shirley went on to explain that she had purchased sneakers, a pair of earrings, and two sweaters. At home, later that night, her mother told her about the murders, which by then were all over the news. "I asked what their names were," Shirley told the investigators. "And she told me 'Harris' and that's when I made the connection."[7]

Continuing her statement, Shirley said that the next day she confronted Michael. She was angry, she said, not only because she thought he had committed the crimes but also because he had involved her in them by lying to her about the source of the credit card. She added that Michael told her that if the police came for him, he would commit suicide. Asked if he threatened her to keep her silent, she replied, "Deep down, I don't think he would have harmed me. But he had said that if any of us went to the police, that we could just forget it. I interpreted that to mean that if anyone told, he would harm me or some member of the family. I told him that if he felt that way, why not come over here and blow me away while I'm sleeping."[8]

While many in the community believed that Michael Kinge had been summarily executed by the police, all the officers involved were exonerated and never charged for their actions. Based on the fingerprint and handwriting evidence, identifications, and her own statement, Shirley was initially charged with murder, arson, and burglary. When it became evident that the state had no evidence that Shirley had been involved in the killings, the murder charge was dropped and she was indicted for burglary, arson, hindering prosecution, criminal possession of stolen property, and forgery.

At her initial court appearances on these charges, the prosecutor, local District Attorney George Dentes, argued against bail for Shirley because of her financial assets and lack of community ties. He even went so far as to push the court to deny her appointment of a lawyer at public expense. Dentes told the court that Shirley, who barely squeaked by on her meager earnings cleaning houses, had "very substantial real estate holdings"[9] that made her ineligible for free counsel. As it turned out, Shirley did own a small undeveloped parcel in the northern Adirondacks. Though worthless as a practical matter, the land was appraised at about 10 to 15 thousand dollars. Bail was set at $50,000, which for Shirley might as well have been $50 million. As for assigned counsel, the court agreed that she was indigent and appointed Ithaca criminal defense lawyer William P. Sullivan to represent her.

Long before I met him, I had heard of Sullivan through other defense attorneys around the state, who marveled at his unparalleled work ethic, fierce devotion to his clients, and uncanny ability to drive prosecutors to the point of distraction. Even in minor criminal matters, Sullivan routinely filed pretrial motions that exceeded a thousand pages, raising and litigating every conceivable legal issue and, in many instances, forcing prosecutors to drop or reduce charges simply because they did not have the time or energy to keep up with his paperwork.

Bill Sullivan reluctantly accepted appointment as Shirley's attorney because, as one of New York's premier criminal defense lawyers, he already had more work than he could reasonably handle. Assigned cases, like Shirley's paid only 25 to 40 dollars an hour, which was peanuts compared with what Sullivan could earn in private-pay cases. But money could not have been an issue in his initial reluctance or his ultimate decision to take Shirley's case; though he would eventually spend thousands of hours on the case, he never even bothered to bill the county a dime for her defense.

Unable to make bail, Shirley sat in the Tompkins County jail for nine months awaiting trial. Shortly before her trial, I served as an expert witness for one of Bill Sullivan's paying clients, a Cornell student charged with date rape. Though the young defendant had been convicted and sentenced to serve two to six years in prison, Sullivan appealed his conviction and it was later overturned. In the course of my work on that case, Sullivan and I discussed Shirley's case. In October 1990, with the trial rapidly approaching, Sullivan petitioned the court to order the county to pay me to conduct a forensic psychological evaluation of the voluntariness of Shirley's statement to the state police.

Under New York state law at that time, an indigent criminal defendant was entitled to have experts and investigators paid for by the county but only up to a total of $300 for all experts and investigators used. I have worked on many cases over the years under this arrangement because to do otherwise would have effectively denied a defendant any access to an expert. I would have accepted such a fee arrangement in this case, if needed, although given the amount of work I eventually put into it, I would have been paid well less than the federal minimum wage.

Fortunately, New York law also allowed assigned counsel such as Bill Sullivan to petition the court to pay an expert more than $300 where the case presented extraordinary circumstances. By any stretch of the imagination, this case was extraordinary, and Sullivan took advantage of that law in asking the court to direct the county to pay me a somewhat more reasonable fee for any work I did on the case. In making his pitch to the court, Sullivan wrote: "The case at bar is an extraordinary case in virtually every respect [including] the estimated million dollar plus expenditures made by the prosecutor, the police authorities and others to try this case."[10] He also argued that the 1965 law limiting an expert's fees to $300 was unconstitutional because enforcing it would effectively deny his client the right to a fair trial. The court avoided ruling on the constitutional issue by quickly granting Sullivan's motion to hire me at a more reasonable but modest fee.

A week later, after reviewing hundreds of pages of witness statements and transcripts from the preliminary hearing, I drove three hours to the Tompkins County Jail and spent the afternoon interviewing Shirley Kinge. The law on confessions is clear: Suspects who are in police custody at the time of interrogation must be warned that they have the right to remain silent, that anything they say can and will be held against them in a court of law, that they have the right to the presence of an attorney during any questioning, and that if they cannot afford a lawyer, the state will pay for one. In addition to these *Miranda* warnings, familiar to anyone who has ever watched a TV cop show, the law requires that unless suspects knowingly, intelligently, and voluntarily waive these rights, any statements they make to the police may not be introduced as evidence. Similarly, the law provides that to be admissible at trial any statement a suspect makes must be shown to have been made voluntarily. And the burden of showing that lies with the prosecution.

Sullivan planned to contest the voluntariness of Shirley's waiver of her rights and the voluntariness of her confession. The confession implicated her only in the criminal use of the Harris credit cards. But as a practical matter, if a jury believed that the statement was voluntarily made, they might also be more likely to believe that Shirley was somehow involved in the burglary and arson. Thus, my purpose in examining Shirley was to determine whether she understood her rights, voluntarily waived them, and voluntarily told the police of her role in using the credit cards.

It has always amazed me that even the smartest suspects will listen to their rights and then talk to the police. After all, the police are telling you flat out that you have a right not to talk to them and that if you do, they will use whatever you say against you. They are as much as telling you to be quiet. No criminal suspect can benefit from talking to the police after having been warned not to, but most cannot keep their mouths shut. Suspects' reasons for talking to the police vary from case to case, but often involve what seems to me to be a deeply ingrained learned drive to respond to allegations of wrongdoing, especially when the allegations are false.

That certainly seemed to be an operative factor in Shirley's case. After reading Shirley her rights, the police repeatedly accused her of doing things she knew she had not done, including starting a fire to cover up the killings. Instead of sitting there in silence or demanding a lawyer, Shirley did what came naturally; she repeatedly denied the allegations.

Even then, however, all the police would have had was a series of denials unless they could somehow break down Shirley's defenses and overcome her will. To understand how easy that was and how it happened, consider what Shirley's life was like in the weeks leading up to the interrogation, what happened to her that morning, and what her mental state was when the police repeatedly accused her of crimes and refused to accept her denials.

Shirley, of course, had good reason to suspect that her son had been involved in a heinous crime and that she, too, might well be in serious trouble for using the Harrises' credit cards. For nearly two weeks prior to her arrest, Shirley was openly followed everywhere by the police.

Then, too, there was the way in which she was arrested. Early in the morning, armed State Police officers wearing bullet-proof vests over plain clothes stormed into her home, burst into her bedroom and confronted her with shouts of "Police! Police! Stay where you are! Show me your hands!"[11] Shirley's first response was to shout, "Don't kill the baby,"[12] referring to her grandson, who was sleeping in a nearby room. One officer asked Shirley where her clothes were. When Shirley pointed to slacks and a sweatshirt, the officer searched them and then told her to get dressed.

Once dressed, Shirley was handcuffed, escorted out of her apartment, placed in a police car, and driven to the State Police barracks in Cortland. At the Cortland barracks, state troopers accused Shirley of being involved in the Harris murders and peppered her with questions but refused to answer hers, especially those she asked about her mother, son and grandson.

"We have reason to believe that you're heavily involved, Mrs. Kinge, in those brutal murders. We want some answers," one of the interrogators told Shirley.[13] Shirley denied any involvement in the crime and kept asking about the whereabouts and condition of Michael. After over two hours of questioning that was obviously going nowhere, the lead investigator decided to play his ace in the hole. Letting Shirley know that her son was dead, he told her he did not know whether Michael had committed suicide or "we killed him."[14] Devastated by the news, Shirley collapsed to the floor, requested to see her son's body, and was falsely told that that was "impossible."[15]

Barely giving Shirley a chance to catch her breath, the police seized on her grief to press their interrogation. Finally, Shirley gave in and acknowledged her role in the credit card fraud. Despite her repeated assertions that she had never even been to the Harris home, much less involved in the killings or the fire, the interrogators continued to push her to confess to murder or at least arson. At one point, one of the officers became agitated and told her, "For Christ's sake, Shirley. We've had four people brutally murdered inside their home. What in the hell do you think you're doing sitting here and telling me lies? I know you were in that house."[16]

Confronted with her fingerprints being found on the gas can at the scene, Shirley told the police that if her prints were on any gas can, it could only be because she had once borrowed such a can from a neighbor when her son's girlfriend ran out of gas.

After reviewing all the relevant documents (which included the police officers' own sworn testimony at the preliminary hearing), interviewing Shirley and listening to her account of the interrogation and the events leading up to it, I concluded that her statement to the police was not voluntary but rather the product of her distraught mental state and the coercive tactics used by the police to overcome her will.

By the time I was called to testify at Shirley's trial, the jury had already heard all of the prosecution's evidence, including the compelling testimony of David Harding, the State Police investigator who had reported discovering Shirley's fingerprints on the gas can found at the crime scene. Harding's testimony was key to the prosecution's case because it was their only means of linking Shirley to the arson and burglary of the Harrises' home.

My evaluation of Shirley was limited to the voluntariness of her confession, but I had given a great deal of thought to the fingerprint evidence. Was Shirley lying about her role in the crimes? Had she actually been there when the Harrises were killed, or at least when the fire was set? Did she try to help her son cover up his monstrous deeds? If so, then what did that say about her truthfulness with me?

As I often explain on the witness stand, I am not a lie detector, but in my professional work I do have to make judgments about the veracity of what people tell me. I readily acknowledge that if someone lies to me, and I base my opinion on what he tells me, then my opinion may be worthless.

Obviously, I had no way of knowing for certain that Shirley Kinge was truthful, but her accounts of the relevant events were consistent and supported by the other evidence I had reviewed—except for the gas can evidence.

I did not see Harding's testimony, but I heard about it at length from Bill Sullivan and the media. Harding was on the witness stand four days offering testimony that supported the version of the case presented by the district attorney in his opening statement. George Dentes, the DA, had told the jury the evidence would show that Shirley had been at the

Harris home on December 23, 1989, that she had poured gasoline on the floor and, in her haste to leave, had "lost her cool, dropped the can and didn't have the time to wipe off her prints."[17]

By all accounts, Harding was an extremely effective and believable witness. There was only one flaw in his testimony, a gap in the evidentiary chain that Sullivan tried to exploit on cross-examination. Harding described the classic process by which he lifted the fingerprints from the can with tape. He then told the jury that after photographing the can and comparing the prints with Shirley's, he wiped the can clean and discarded the fingerprint tape. As Sullivan made clear, that meant that no one else could corroborate Harding's findings and thus all the jury had to go on was Harding's word, his sworn testimony.

As Sullivan also made clear to anyone who would listen, he thought Harding was a liar. The problem was that thinking was one thing, proving was something else. I was skeptical and even contacted my brother, a veteran police detective in a nearby city, to inquire (without revealing why) about Harding's reputation. My brother was effusive in his praise of the State Police investigator. Harding, he said, was a rising star, and his brilliant forensic work had cracked a number of difficult cases.

Years later, I would learn that not everyone shared my brother's opinion of David Harding. Indeed, when Harding's boss, Senior Investigator David McElligott, heard of Harding's testimony about wiping the can and discarding the tape, he told Dentes, the district attorney, "I'm beginning to believe there's something rotten about Harding, and that maybe the woman was never in the house."[18]

When the time came for me to testify—nearly four months into the longest trial in the county's history, a trial that would ultimately include 116 witnesses—I was surprised to learn that the trial was being broadcast gavel-to-gavel by a local TV channel and was being covered by the national media. Live television coverage of trials in New York state has since been banned out of fear that witnesses might feel intimidated. I have testified in numerous televised trials around the country, including this one, and can honestly say that the presence of the camera in the courtroom had no effect on me. But then, I never have anything riding on the outcome of the cases in which I testify. I get paid regardless of who wins and loses, and unlike the judge and the DA, I don't have to stand for reelection.

In Shirley Kinge's trial, though, it seemed clear to me that the cameras had a profound effect on at least some of the key players. The courtroom was much more formal than usual, and the lawyers and judge seemed keenly aware that their every move was being watched by members of the community, many of whom had made it clear that the death of Michael Kinge was not enough payback for the brutal murders of the Harrises.

My testimony was fairly simple but complex in its explanation. Shirley's statement was not voluntary because when she was arrested she was on the verge of a mental breakdown and was pushed over the edge by the police report that they had killed her son. In my view, the police had taken advantage of Shirley's distraught mental state through the use of isolation, physical and psychological control, withholding of information, and intimidation.

Before I had the chance to fully explain my expert opinion to the jury, Dentes objected, claiming that my testimony wasn't needed because the lay jurors were capable of figuring out for themselves whether Shirley's statement was voluntary. Sullivan countered that the psychology of confessions is well beyond the ken of a lay jury and that courts elsewhere in the state had accepted this kind of expert testimony. Indeed, I had frequently given such testimony in cases in New York and other states.

The judge asked for an offer of proof. What more, he wanted to know, would I be telling the jury? Outside the jury's hearing but on the record, Sullivan and I informed the judge that my opinion was based on numerous facts. Shirley, a 55-year-old black woman, had been forcibly removed from her home and family at the crack of dawn by heavily armed but nonuniformed white strangers who literally stormed into her house, rousted her half-naked from bed, forced her to dress in front of two men, told her what clothing she could and could not wear, refused to allow her to take any identification with her, handcuffed her, forced her into a car where she was surrounded by three plain-clothed officers, drove her to the State Police station in another city rather the one close to her home, refused to tell her where she was being taken, why or what was going to happen there, and refused to respond to her questions about the whereabouts and safety of her mother, son, and grandson.

On arrival in Cortland, the police introduced themselves using their formal titles but repeatedly referred to Shirley by her first name. While the police refused to answer any of Shirley's questions, they demanded repeatedly that she answer theirs. Though Shirley tried to remain strong and refused to cooperate despite hours of interrogation, the police continued to grill her and finally resorted to telling her of the death of her son. That revelation triggered a natural grief response and led Shirley to become hysterical. The police response to Shirley's mental breakdown was not to call a physician or mental health professional, but to offer her a roll of toilet paper and a glass of water.

The effect of all this, I explained, was to distort Shirley's perception, alter her ability to control her behavior, impair her cognitive capacities such as memory and the ability to reason, and even alter her bodily functions as evidenced by her increased thirst and frequent need to urinate.

After considering what I had to say, the judge ruled that the jury could not hear the rest of my testimony, a ruling that set off a firestorm at the courthouse and triggered charges of misconduct against Shirley's lawyer, Bill Sullivan. Following the judge's limitation of my testimony, Sullivan and I left the courtroom and were met by a number of reporters who questioned us about what they had just observed either on TV or in the courtroom. As one reporter described it, "William P. Sullivan Jr., Kinge's attorney, said muzzling Ewing dealt a lethal blow to his defense."[19]

When segments of Sullivan's comments were aired that night on a local television station, District Attorney Dentes filed a formal compliant with the state bar authorities, alleging that the defense attorney had violated the lawyer's Code of Professional Responsibility "in that, while representing a criminal defendant in a felony jury trial, he made extrajudicial statements in a live television broadcast which he knew or reasonably should have known would have a substantial likelihood of materially prejudicing the proceeding."[20]

Whether my full testimony would have made a difference will never be known. In hindsight, my own suspicion is that it would not have made much of a difference. Michael Kinge was dead, and the community still wanted blood. Dentes's response to the claim that Shirley's confession was not voluntary was that Shirley had gone into the interrogation with two plans. One, he said was, "nobody talks, everybody walks."[21] The second plan, he argued, was to blame everything on her son. "She was never broken; she was never coerced," he told the jury. "She told as much as she wanted to tell."[22]

Dentes also relied heavily on the one solid piece of evidence that Shirley not only engaged in credit card fraud but had been part of the earlier crime, at least the arson. In his closing statement, he repeatedly reminded the jury of the evidence that neither my testimony nor anyone else's could have rebutted: Shirley's fingerprints on the gas can found at the crime scene. Despite the private doubts about this particular piece of evidence expressed to him earlier by Harding's boss, Dentes boldly told the jury, "The defendant left her calling card, by which I mean her fingerprints. The rock-hard core, the terra firma, is that her fingerprints were on the gas can. There's no innocent explanation."[23]

After a day of deliberation, the jury convicted Shirley on all counts. In a press conference on the courthouse steps—much like the one Bill Sullivan had given when the judge refused to let the jury hear all of my testimony—Dentes celebrated Shirley's convictions and pointed to David Harding, who stood next to him, as a hero.

Shirley Kinge did not regard Harding as a hero. In fact, two months later as she faced the court for sentencing, she made it clear what she thought of him. Shirley admitted having used the stolen credit card and said she accepted whatever punishment the court might impose for that crime. But, addressing the arson and burglary charges, Shirley told the judge, "During the trial, the prosecutor called several witnesses who were loose with the truth. One of these witnesses flat out lied about fingerprints, about conversations with me and about other things, like wiping the can clean to make it shine."[24] As for Dentes, Shirley said, "He did everything he could to keep the truth away from the jury."[25]

The judge was unimpressed by Shirley's articulate statement. He imposed the maximum sentence allowed by law: 15 to 30 years in prison. Under the judge's order, Shirley would be over 70 years old before she was even eligible to be considered for parole. However, given the heinous nature of the crimes involved, it was likely that she would never be paroled and would instead die in prison.

Dentes struck me as a sore winner. He continued to press his complaint against Bill Sullivan, and it took a New York appeals court to decide that the defense attorney had done nothing wrong. As the court concluded:

> [Sullivan's] television interview was a mere drop in the ocean of publicity surrounding this trial, and indeed, all of the matters remarked upon by [him] had been otherwise publicized prior to the interview. For example . . . *The Ithaca Journal* and *The Post-Standard* in Syracuse both carried prominent articles detailing the testimony given by Dr. Ewing in court, in the absence of the jury, which the trial court disallowed. While we acknowledge that a public extrajudicial statement by a defense attorney generally carries more authoritative weight than media publicity [Sullivan's] brief interview, given during the publicity-saturated circumstances of this trial, was not of a kind to so qualitatively alter public knowledge or mood that he should have known it would carry a substantial likelihood of materially prejudicing the proceeding.[26]

While Shirley began serving her sentence at the Bedford Hills Correctional Facility, outside New York City, Bill Sullivan was assigned by the court to appeal Shirley's convictions. In New York, as in most states, the appellate process is long and complex. It would not have been unheard of for Shirley's appeal to have taken several years before it was even heard, much less ruled on. Meanwhile, having been convicted, rightly or wrongly, she would sit behind bars.

While the wheels of New York appellate justice were slowly grinding in the Kinge case, David Harding, who had been awarded a State Police commendation for his outstanding work on the case, decided to make a career move. His plan was to leave the New York State Police and use his newly minted credentials as a hero to join the Central

Intelligence Agency. As part of the screening process for employment as a CIA agent, Harding underwent routine polygraph testing on January 14, 1991, just two months after Shirley had been convicted. The polygraph examiner asked Harding if he had ever violated the law. Harding candidly replied that he had stolen a bicycle when he was a child, stolen money from his employer before he became a State Police officer, stolen money that was to have been used in a State Police drug sting operation, and added or subtracted weight from drugs seized from dealers to make the charges more or less serious. More important, Harding told the CIA polygrapher that on numerous occasions he had falsified fingerprint evidence against criminal suspects to help secure convictions.

To repeat, that was on *January 14, 1991*. Not surprisingly, Harding was not hired by the CIA. Instead, he kept his position with the New York State Police, though he missed a lot of work, claiming a questionable back injury. It was not until *May 26, 1992,* 16 months after Harding's CIA polygraph, that federal agents notified New York State Police officials of even the barest outline of what Harding had told the polygraph examiner. Even then, the New York officers could not be given any specific details until they received federal security clearances, a process that took over two weeks. Meanwhile, with no inkling of what was happening, Shirley Kinge went about her daily routine as an inmate at Bedford Hills, waiting for her appeal and knowing that she had been wrongfully convicted but having no way to prove it.

Harding's response was that none of what he'd told the CIA was true. He had made it all up, he said to show them that he was the kind of applicant who could be counted on to do the CIA's dirty work. "They weren't looking for choir boys or Boy Scouts," he told the State Police internal affairs officer who eventually questioned him.[27]

News of Harding's imminent fall from grace traveled fast. When the word reached Bill Sullivan, he immediately demanded a new trial for Shirley. Dentes resisted, noting that so far there had been no clear evidence that Harding faked the fingerprint evidence in the Kinge case. He also pointed out that even if Harding had faked the evidence and Shirley were to be exonerated, she could not complain about the time she was serving because she would still be guilty of credit card fraud. "There won't be any apology from me, that's for sure," the district attorney said. "It's not like she's a totally innocent person sitting in the can."[28]

Harding was soon charged and initially appeared before Judge Betty Friedlander. I had met Judge Friedlander during the first case I did with Bill Sullivan, the Cornell date rape prosecution. Friedlander, whom I later came to know personally, presided over that trial, and was as tough a judge as I had ever met. She certainly cut me no slack but at least allowed me to testify fully. Later, when she left the bench because of her age, she returned to practicing law and called on me to evaluate a couple of her clients.

Judge Friedlander felt strongly that a special prosecutor should be appointed to handle the case against David Harding because she saw the obvious. Allowing Dentes to prosecute Harding would create at least the appearance of a conflict of interests. After all, Harding had been Dentes's star witness against Shirley, and the DA had hailed him as a hero. Dentes resisted Judge Friedlander's move to appoint a special prosecutor. Over his objections, the judge ordered Dentes off the case and appointed a local attorney to serve as independent counsel for the state. As evidence of what she called "manifest inroads in the District Attorney's neutrality,"[29] the judge cited Dentes's recommendation that Harding be released on his own recognizance rather then being required to post any bail.

At the hearing on Shirley Kinge's request for a new trial, Dentes made another remarkable argument. He told the court that Harding's admission to having falsified evidence in another case unrelated to the Kinge prosecution presented sufficient newly discovered evidence to warrant a retrial for Shirley, but refused to concede that Harding had testified falsely in her first trial.

Despite Dentes's legal tap dance, the judge really had no choice but to grant a new trial. On September 11, 1992, after having been locked up for more than two and a half years, Shirley was released on $25,000 bail to await her second trial.

Fortunately for Shirley, there never was another trial. The special prosecutor, who replaced Dentes, uncovered 34 criminal cases in which Harding and fellow State Police officers tampered with evidence against criminal defendants and/or committed perjury at their trials. The prosecutor also reported that Harding admitted cutting a section out of the floorboard in Michael Kinge's apartment after his fellow state police officers killed Kinge. Harding told the special counsel that he was attempting to hide evidence of what he thought was an unjustified shooting.

In a plea deal in which Harding agreed to provide evidence against other crooked State Police officers and come clean about all the evidence they had falsified, he pled guilty to four counts of first-degree perjury, including having lied under oath about finding Shirley Kinge's prints on the gas can.

At sentencing, Harding had the audacity to paint what he had done to Shirley and other criminal defendants as a service to the community. The admitted perjurer told Judge Friedlander, "In these cases where I have acted unethically, it is because of certainty by myself and others that the defendant was dangerous to the public and should be removed from society. I never acted with bad intent, nor did I do so for personal gain. My reward was simply the protection of the public, wherein my own family resides."[30]

When the special prosecutor who had finally brought Harding to justice heard these remarks, he was "astonished."[31] "My jaw dropped when he said that," the prosecutor said. "It's quite clear he hasn't gotten the message yet."[32]

Apparently, Judge Friedlander concluded that Harding was "dangerous to the public and should be removed from society."[33] Lamenting that the law could not adequately sanction Harding because "there isn't a crime in the book for willfully destroying or attempting to destroy public confidence in its criminal justice system,"[34] the judge sentenced Harding to serve 4 to 12 years in prison and pay a $10,000 fine.

Harding later received the same sentence for similar crimes committed in another county where the sentencing judge told him, "You had it all. You had education, you had intelligence, you hold a master's degree. But you are so stupid that you can't begin to comprehend the highest concept of American law enforcement. And that is that no man is above the law. The sad thing is, I don't think you'll ever understand what you did."[35] As part of Harding's original plea bargain, the sentences from both counties were to run concurrently, meaning that Harding could be released after serving no more than four years.

In the wake of Harding's admissions, the investigation of evidence tampering and police perjury was broadened and eventually led to the convictions of four other state police officers and the resignations of two of their superiors.

As for Shirley, she was finally vindicated two years to the day after her convictions. On November 16, 1992, she pled guilty to misdemeanor forgery for illegally using the Harrises' credit card. The burglary and arson charges were dismissed. She received the sentence that she probably would have received originally had it not been for Harding's misconduct: a one-year conditional discharge and an order to make restitution in the amount of $635 to the stores she defrauded.

Amazingly, but perhaps not surprisingly, David Harding served only the minimum sentence, four years, before the New York state parole board released him.

CHAPTER 6

Child Abuse Victim, Sexual Predator, or Both?

6

The June 1988 graduation ceremony at LaSalle High School in Niagara Falls was unique in the school's long history. Never before had the class valedictorian failed to show up and give a speech to the graduating class and their families. This time, though, the top student in the class was missing for a devastating reason—just hours earlier, he had been arrested and jailed on a murder charge.

Few were surprised that William "Billy" Shrubsall was the number one student in his high school class of 250 students. He had a superior IQ and had been a straight-A student for most of his life. At 17, he was also handsome and articulate well beyond his years, had served as editor of the high school yearbook, and was a standout in chorus, drama, math club, and student council. During his senior year, Billy had been accepted by and offered scholarships to a host of top colleges, including the University of Pennsylvania and the University of Chicago. His ultimate goal was to attend Harvard Law School.

At the same time, few if any of those who knew him would have predicted that Billy would ever be charged with murder, much less on the eve of his graduation. Neighbors and friends knew him as a polite and respectful, though perhaps somewhat spoiled, only child from a solid working-class family, who had never before been in trouble with the law. And, if they were surprised to learn of his arrest, they were astounded to learn the grisly nature of his crime.

In the early morning hours of June 25, 1988, less than 12 hours before Billy was to deliver the valedictory address and receive his diploma, he ran to the home of a neighbor crying for help. His mother, he said, had been attacked by two male intruders and severely beaten. When Niagara Falls police officers arrived at the Shrubsall's modest but well-kept brick bungalow minutes later, they discovered the 300-pound body of 56-year-old Mariane "Marge" Shrubsall lying in a hallway, beaten beyond recognition. Her corpse, the floor beneath it, and the walls above it were splattered with blood.

Confronted about the crimson splotches on his clothing, Billy claimed that he had unsuccessfully tried to protect his mother from her assailants. The police were skeptical, and within a few hours Billy confessed to killing his mother. The autopsy indicated that she had been struck some 20 times with a blunt instrument, but Billy claimed he had killed his mother in self-defense. For years, he said, particularly since the death of his father in 1985, she had abused him verbally and physically.

While his father had been an easygoing and supportive man who encouraged Billy's participation in sports, his mother had seen him as a kind of intellectual project through which she could raise her own flagging self-esteem. From Billy's infancy on, Marge had responded to his obvious intellectual gifts by relentlessly pushing him to achieve. Under her tutelage, Billy read by age two, knew the multiplication tables by three, played the guitar and identified the works of major composers by five, and understood algebra and geometry by seven. Yet, for all his academic accomplishments, nothing Billy could ever do pleased Marge; even straight-A grades weren't enough to convince her that he was doing his best at school. Why, she would often ask, had he not gotten the highest grade of all?

Later—after Billy's father died and Billy began to struggle with the biological and psychological imperatives of adolescence—his perceived "failures" were met with physical violence. When Billy displeased Marge or failed to meet her demands for perfection, she responded by beating him with her fists and various household objects. Just a week before the killing, Billy told police, his mother had beaten him with a towel bar because he'd arrived home seven minutes after his curfew.

On the night of the killing, Billy had arrived home after his mother was asleep, and the killing might never have occurred had his girlfriend not called him to say that he had left his watch at her house. After a quick phone conversation, Billy walked to the girl's home to retrieve his watch and some photos he had also left behind. When he returned home, 15 to 30 minutes later, it was nearly 1:00 AM. Marge was awake and enraged, ready to head out in the car looking for her son. She yelled at Billy for about two hours, told him she planned to call his girlfriend's parents and tell them their daughter was a "slut," threatened him, and eventually attacked him.[1] As Billy told the police several hours later, his mother became increasingly enraged, denounced him as "slime" and a "son of a bitch," struck him repeatedly, threatened to kill him, and finally backed him into his bedroom, where he grabbed a wooden baseball bat and beat her to death.[2]

Asked by one of the detectives why he had lied to the neighbors about what happened, Billy replied, "I was just hoping that people didn't have to know that she beats me. I didn't want that to happen to her name, and I didn't want it to happen to my name. I just didn't want it to happen."[3]

Though Billy spent his graduation day in jail, he was soon released on bail posted by his mother's sister, who also put up the money to hire a top-flight criminal lawyer, Paul Cleary. In recent years, Cleary had represented several high-profile homicide defendants in the western New York area. One was Leslie Emick, a battered woman who shot her abusive common-law husband to death while he slept. Another was Ronald Longmire, an African American college student who, when surrounded in his dormitory room by a throng of angry and threatening white youths, stabbed one of them to death with a kitchen knife. I served as an expert witness for the defense in the Longmire case, and to the surprise of many, the young defendant was found not guilty.

Paul Cleary had been referred to me in his defense of Ronnie Longmire by a former student of mine who knew of a concept I had recently developed and written a book about: psychological self-defense. Typically, the law recognizes self-defense as a legal justification for homicide only where, at the time of the killing, the killer reasonably believed that he or she was in imminent danger of death or serious bodily injury at the hands of the person killed. Strict application of that legal doctrine has resulted in the conviction of many women and children who have killed their abusive husbands or parents because such killings often take place when the abuser is asleep or otherwise preoccupied, not engaged in domestic violence. Under the proposed doctrine of psychological self-defense, which I detailed in a book called *Battered Women Who Kill,* a killing would be justified if committed to protect oneself from an imminent threat of "extremely serious psychological injury . . . that significantly limits the meaning and value of one's physical existence."[4]

Both Ronnie Longmire and Billy Shrubsall killed in the course of physical confrontations with their victims. In neither case was the concept of "psychological self-defense" a real issue. Still, given that neither case neatly fit within the parameters of self-defense law, in both cases, Paul Cleary was looking for a psychological expert who might explain to a skeptical jury why his clients' actions ought to be considered justified as self-defense.

Cleary's job as an attorney was to advocate for the best possible outcome for Billy Shrubsall. He knew from his work with me in the Longmire case that my role was not that of advocate but rather one of objective evaluator. As a forensic psychologist, I review the evidence, examine the individual in question, and offer an opinion that may or may not be helpful. Indeed, most of the time, my opinions are not helpful to those who seek and pay for them. Nevertheless, once he was retained, Paul Cleary immediately turned to me to evaluate his new client.

Less than two weeks after killing his mother, Billy Shrubsall sat in my office and, over the course of two days, faced seven hours of questioning much more intense than that he had experienced with the police. Not that I was hostile or particularly harsh, just demanding. The police interrogation, if it could be called such, resulted in a 44-page transcript that was virtually a monologue by the 17-year-old murder suspect. After advising Billy of his *Miranda* rights, the two detectives asked no more than a handful of questions, most of which seemed meant to keep Billy talking and let him know that they were still listening. The questions I posed to Billy covered his entire life, not just the night of the killing. My questions about the killing were detailed and required specific answers, not the sorts of generalities he had given the police.

After examining Billy and reviewing the evidence in the case, I reported my conclusions to his attorney. Soon the case took an unexpected turn. With Cleary's consent, the prosecutors asked me to testify before the grand jury that was called to weigh the evidence against Billy and indict him. I have evaluated thousands of criminal defendants and have testified in over 600 trials, but in only three cases have I been called to testify before a grand jury.

The reason for that is simple. Grand jury proceedings are controlled totally by prosecutors. They decide what witnesses to call, what questions to ask, and what indictments to seek. There is no judge, no defendant and no defense lawyer present, just the prosecutor, the witness, a stenographer, and 23 grand jurors who take their marching orders from the prosecutor. Sol Wachtler, former chief judge of New York's highest court, the Court of Appeals, once complained publicly that prosecutors have so much influence on grand juries that they could get them to "indict a ham sandwich."[5]

Wachtler's candid views were validated by the grand jury proceedings in the well-known case of Bernhard Goetz, the New York vigilante who shot four young black men on one of the city's subway trains two days before Christmas in 1984. Goetz, a mild-mannered electrical engineer, was eventually acquitted of attempted murder. When, immediately after the shootings, public sentiment favored Goetz, the prosecutors got the grand jury to throw out the attempted murder charges and indict Goetz only for illegal possession of a gun. Later, when the tide of public opinion turned against Goetz, prosecutors took the case back to the grand jury and secured a multiple-count attempted murder indictment. In the end, however, a jury acquitted Goetz and convicted him only of illegal possession of a gun.

In inviting and preparing me to testify in the Shrubsall case, the prosecutors were clearly sympathetic to the young defendant who, like Goetz, seemed to be getting a lot of favorable press. I felt certain that the prosecutors did not want Billy indicted for murder, but preferred that he be indicted for some lesser charge such as manslaughter. With that result, they could satisfy the public's demand for criminal accountability and yet show mercy to an apparently abused teenager who everyone agreed had a very bright future that would be destroyed by a lengthy prison sentence.

After meeting at length with the prosecutors—both of whom seemed sincere in their desire to do justice in this case—I testified about Billy's history of being physically and psychologically abused by his mother. I explained how the abuse had begun early in his life but had escalated rapidly after his father died. I also detailed the pathological relationship between Billy and Marge, who viewed herself as a failure and lived vicariously through her son and his many accomplishments. Finally, I tried to explain how that relationship had culminated in her death:

> She felt like she was a failure all her life. You've got a superstar, you can see the temptation to live your life through your child. . . . She was watching herself lose control of a person she had control of for 18 years, a person she created and made. This woman was a person whose life was about to be emptied. He was her life. She had nothing else. And she snapped. . . . Beating [his] mother's head in was 16 years of pent-up emotion exploding at the end of a baseball bat. The floodgate broke.[6]

If, as I suspected, the prosecutors were hoping that my testimony might give the jury reason to indict Billy for manslaughter rather than (or in addition to) murder, they got at least part of their wish. The grand jury returned indictments for both murder and manslaughter. In New York, what would otherwise be murder may be charged as first-degree manslaughter if, at the time of the killing, the perpetrator was in a state of extreme emotional disturbance for which there was a reasonable cause or explanation. My testimony made it clear not only that Billy was in such a state when he pummeled his mother with the bat but that his state of mind had a reasonable cause or explanation: 16 years of abuse.

Once the grand jury indicted Billy for both murder and manslaughter, the road was paved for a plea bargain. Convicted of murder, he could have been sentenced to 25 years to life in prison. Guilty of manslaughter, he could serve from $8\frac{1}{3}$ to 25 years, but would be eligible for youthful offender status. Under New York law at that time, a defendant younger than 19 could be adjudicated a youthful offender if he were found guilty of or pleaded guilty to a charge other than murder and had no prior criminal record. That decision—which would not only expunge Billy's criminal record but limit his punishment to a sentence of 16 months to four years in prison—lay in the discretion of the sentencing judge.

With the prosecutor's consent, if not encouragement, Billy pleaded guilty to manslaughter and went before Judge Charles Hannigan for sentencing. Popularly known as "Hangman Hannigan," the county judge was a no-nonsense jurist with a penchant for defying expectations. For example, 15 convictions in his court were overturned on appeal because he insisted on giving juries his own definition of "reasonable doubt," a definition the appeals court repeatedly said was wrong. True to his nickname, Hannigan declined to grant Billy youthful offender status and sentenced him instead to 5 to 15 years in adult prison. At sentencing, Hannigan told Billy he did not believe that the boy had been abused and said, "Show me a kid that hasn't been spanked, hit, walloped, I'll show you a spoiled kid."[7]

But Hannigan did not have the final word in the matter. The judge, whose idiosyncratic "reasonable doubt" instructions had been soundly rejected by his superiors on the appellate bench, was soon overruled. After reviewing the matter, the same appeals court held 4–1 that Hannigan had erred in denying Billy youthful offender status. Citing the circumstances surrounding the crime and Billy's exemplary prior record, the court found that his prospects for rehabilitation were excellent. The court also noted:

> [S]ignificant mitigating circumstances exist in that defendant presented evidence to the sentencing court that he was an abused child and that the act he committed arose out of that fact. Dr. Charles Ewing, a psychologist, testified at the Grand Jury and reported to the sentencing court his opinion that defendant had been abused, both psychologically and physically, by the victim. We consider it to be particularly significant that defendant's aunt, the victim's sister, wrote to the sentencing court on defendant's behalf. Having observed the dynamics within this family for years, she opined that "the abuses of years culminated in the terrible act that Billy committed: that he just exploded with rage." Moreover, the sentencing court acknowledged that defendant's act was not premeditated.[8]

As a result of the appellate court's decision, Billy's criminal record was expunged and he was resentenced to one and one-third to four years in prison. While incarcerated, he had no disciplinary problems, completed assigned programs, worked on college courses, volunteered as a teacher's aide, and served as a peer counselor. In part because of his good conduct in prison, Billy served the minimum sentence and was paroled after 16 months behind bars. He remained on parole for another year and a half, but his parole supervision was terminated early because he was considered a "stellar parolee."[9]

When Billy was released from prison, parole authorities referred him for counseling. But after just two sessions, mental health professionals at a local psychiatric facility refused to provide Billy with ongoing psychotherapy because they concluded that he posed no danger to himself or others.

Once out of prison, Billy resumed his education, graduating from the Ivy League's University of Pennsylvania. After briefly selling cars and working in a Niagara Falls restaurant, he found a job as a stock analyst on Wall Street.

Had the story of Billy Shrubsall and the law ended there, it would have been one of the criminal justice system's great triumphs and the source of significant satisfaction for me, Paul Cleary, the prosecutors, the appeals court, and the many others who hoped Billy would succeed despite what had been done to him and what he had done in response. But, sadly, the Shrubsall saga was far from over.

On January 6, 1995, a young woman was driving on Interstate-90, the New York State Thruway, when she was pulled over by a man in an unmarked car. The man told her he was a police officer. He said he intended to write her up for a traffic infraction but that she could avoid the ticket by giving him oral sex. The woman fled but managed to get the "officer's" license plate number. Following up on the plate number, police soon learned that the man was William Shrubsall. Shrubsall admitted pulling the woman over but claimed he wanted to tell her that there was something wrong with her car. He denied claiming to be a police officer or asking for sex. Although the police charged Shrubsall with felony impersonation of a police officer, the charges were dropped when the woman, on learning the identity of the perpetrator, said she was too frightened to testify.

Three months later, Shrubsall was back in police custody, arrested this time for grabbing a woman's buttocks as she walked down a major commercial street wearing stereo headphones. Convicted of sexual abuse, Shrubsall served 60 days in the county jail.

Barely out of confinement, Shrubsall struck again. In August 1995, he was arrested for sexually abusing a 17-year-old girl who had gotten drunk and fallen asleep at a house party. Authorities alleged that Shrubsall had provided the girl with alcohol and then, once she was drunk, tried to force her to give him oral sex, masturbated, and ejaculated on her face as she lay unconscious. Faced with charges that could land him in prison for years, Shrubsall was again bailed out by his aunt, who posted $20,000 for his release pending trial and allowed him to stay in her home.

In May 1996, Shrubsall went to trial before Charles Hannigan, the judge who had earlier denied him youthful offender status and never believed that Shrubsall had been abused by his mother. On the day that his attorney and the prosecutor were to complete their closing arguments to the jury, Shrubsall disappeared, leaving a handwritten note in his aunt's home. The apparent suicide note read in part:

> Let's face it, losing means the next eight-and-one-third-to-25 years are spoken for. Years filled with rapes at the hands of HIV-infected inmates and frequent stabbings (probable death) as an accused sex offender. It is all my fault I lost for two reasons: (1) because I allowed myself to set foot in this awful county again after graduation, and (2) because I agreed not to testify. I was a liar and a deceiver, and a "sexual predator" because I could not prove otherwise having stood mute. I have nothing: no family (except for you), no friends, no girlfriend or wife, no money, no job, no prospects, meaningless education and mountains of debt. Most of all, no hope. I meant to do this earlier, but I haven't had the guts. So tonight I got drunk and walked down to the Falls. To my knowledge, no one has ever survived the American Falls. I don't think I will either.[10]

Others, including me, were left to ponder whether Shrubsall actually committed suicide. The consensus among law enforcement officers was that he had simply jumped bail and written the note to cover his tracks. To begin with, his attorney, Christopher Privateer, an experienced and perceptive public defender, told the media that Shrubsall had seemed upbeat rather than depressed during the trial. Privateer said Shrubsall played an active role in his own defense and that at the end of court the day of his disappearance, he told the defense attorney he would see him in court the next morning. Though I had no involvement in the case at that point and declined to respond to the media requests for my speculation, I privately shared the prevailing view that Shrubsall had not thrown himself over Niagara Falls or otherwise committed suicide.

Acting on the intuition that Shrubsall had absconded rather than killed himself, police pleaded with the community for tips that would lead them to the fugitive. Still, the lead investigator from the State Police, was not hopeful. He told the media, "Until he gets into trouble again, he'll be hard to find. He doesn't want to be found, for one thing, and he's not a stupid person."[11]

In any event, whatever had happened to Shrubsall, he never returned to court, his aunt lost the $20,000 bail she had posted for him, the jury found him guilty, and, in November 1996, he was sentenced *in absentia* to seven years in prison. Some of Shrubsall's former classmates reported seeing him in a Niagara Falls bar just a couple of weeks after he disappeared. I seriously doubted such reports because I was convinced that Shrubsall was much too intelligent and resourceful to expose himself to capture so easily.

Although authorities would not know it until nearly two years later, Shrubsall was not in Niagara Falls when his classmates and others claimed to have seen him. In fact, within a day of disappearing from Niagara Falls in May 1996, Shrubsall turned up a thousand miles away in the Canadian city of Halifax, Nova Scotia, staying at a $20 a night shelter for homeless men and filing a welfare application under the alias of Ian Thor Greene. The city of Niagara Falls, of course, immediately borders Canada, and at that time identification was rarely required for Americans entering our neighbor to the north. So it is likely that after leaving his phony suicide note, Shrubsall immediately crossed the border and very quickly made his way to Halifax. The short time frame and his obvious need to travel incognito suggest that he probably traveled by train and/or bus and that he had planned his escape well in advance.

After living for about a month in the Halifax shelter, known as Metro Turning Point, Shrubsall was offered a rental room in the home of Daisy McGuire, who worked at the shelter. Shrubsall lived there for almost a year, working and posing as a college student. McGuire evicted Shrubsall in June 1997 when she learned that he had been arrested for soliciting an undercover police officer posing as a prostitute, fingerprinted, and fined one hundred dollars. Had Canadian authorities run Shrubsall's fingerprints or even bothered to check his record while they briefly had him in custody, they might have learned that the man calling himself Ian Thor Greene was in fact William Chandler Shrubsall, a fugitive from justice. But since his crime was considered minor, no check was done.

Having narrowly escaped capture, Shrubsall changed his cover story and moved into a rented room in the *Sigma Chi* fraternity house at Dalhousie University in Halifax. There he told his fellow residents that he was a 19-year-old premedical student from the Yukon, that his father had died in a car accident and that his mother had met her death in a fire caused by falling asleep while smoking in bed. To maintain the ruse, Shrubsall attended classes and helped a number of the fraternity brothers with their studies. He supported himself by working as a telemarketer, salesman, janitor, and fast food worker. Acquaintances later described Shrubsall as charming and bright, but few believed he was 19 years old or that he was an orphan from the Yukon.

In 1998, Shrubsall embarked on what can fairly be described as a reign of terror on Halifax women. In February, he entered a clothing store and clubbed a 25-year-old female clerk with a baseball bat, shattering her skull and driving shards of bone into her brain. The attack was so vicious that it left the woman unconscious, amnesic, and so severely injured that surgeons needed to place a dozen metal plates and some 50 screws in her head to ensure her survival.

On May 4, 1998, in broad daylight and while being observed by people in nearby homes, Shrubsall chased a 19-year-old woman down a city street, grabbed her from behind, placed her in a choke hold, pulled her into a driveway, stripped her of most of her clothing, pounded her face into the pavement, masturbated on her and stole her backpack and wallet. The woman's face was so badly damaged in the attack that her contact lenses had to be surgically removed.

But what finally led to Shrubsall's legal downfall was a June 22, 1998 attack on a woman he had met in a Halifax nightclub and invited to a party at the fraternity house. As the 26-year-old woman would quickly learn, there was no party. Once she was in Shrubsall's room, he grabbed her and tried to kiss her. When she resisted his advances, he grabbed, punched, and choked her. The altercation spilled into the hallway outside Shrubsall's room, and several other tenants responded to see him on top of the woman, choking her with both hands. Shrubsall then dragged the young woman back into his room by her ankles, locked the door and refused entry to the onlookers, yelling, "Everything is under control."[12] Neighbors, hearing the woman cry, "Help me. He's trying to kill me," located a master key and burst into the room.[13] The woman—who was bruised and bloodied and wearing only panties—ran to her rescuers while Shrubsall grabbed a few belongings and fled by way of a fire escape.

Within a day, police located Shrubsall and arrested him as Ian Thor Greene. DNA testing done on Shrubsall's clothing revealed traces of the woman's blood. A search of his room at the fraternity house turned up the backpack and wallet taken from the woman he assaulted on May 4 and the wallet belonging to the woman he attacked with a baseball bat in February. DNA testing done on Shrubsall's clothing revealed traces of blood containing the DNA of both these victims. DNA testing of the semen found on the clothing of the May 4 victim revealed that it had come from Shrubsall.

At that time, the police were not aware that Ian Thor Greene was actually William Chandler Shrubsall. Indeed, even after a month of questioning him, Canadian authorities had no idea who their suspect was. No idea, that is, until they aired his photograph on Canadian television, and portions of those broadcasts were carried by an American network. Almost immediately, viewers in Niagara Falls contacted the police to tell them that Greene was actually the fugitive Shrubsall.

Though his trial was delayed numerous times by various appeals, Shrubsall was eventually convicted of aggravated sexual assault and robbery. Prosecutors then sought to have Shrubsall adjudicated a dangerous offender, a classification in Canadian law that would put a serial sex offender behind bars for an indeterminate sentence, possibly life.

Prosecutors were so determined to see Shrubsall put away for good that they initiated an investigation that would eventually cost the provincial government approximately half a million dollars. Leaving no stone unturned, the prosecution team found evidence that the crimes for which Shrubsall had been convicted were merely the tip of the iceberg and that his crimes against women had begun well before he beat his mother to death.

To begin with, Canadian officials located a woman who testified that in January 1986 (two years before Marge Shrubsall was killed), when she was 14 years old, she was pushed to the ground by a teenage male, who told her he had a knife, kissed her, and demanded oral sex. She screamed loudly, and her attacker fled. Months later, she said, she identified Shrubsall (a fellow student at her school) as her assailant, based on his distinctive voice and the clothes he was wearing. Instead of reporting the incident to the police, however, the girl said she had her boyfriend assault Shrubsall.

Two other witnesses, women who had been secretaries at a university in Niagara Falls when a 15-year-old Shrubsall attended a summer basketball camp there, testified that Shrubsall had stalked them. According to their testimony, they were middle-aged at the time. Shrubsall, they testified, followed them on campus, chased them, and uttered, "I want you" and "Turn around and you'll change your mind."[14] One of the women testified that when she was stalked, Shrubsall "had this stern kind of look in his eyes, very intense.... I thought at one point that he hates women."[15] She added, "I said there must be something wrong with this guy to be chasing a woman old enough to be his mother."[16]

These incidents were reported to campus police, who referred the allegations to the camp coach when the women agreed not to press charges if Shrubsall received psychiatric treatment. One woman testified that Shrubsall broke down in tears and pleaded with the coach not to inform his mother of the incidents.

Whether Marge Shrubsall ever learned of these allegations is unknown, but at least one other person told her that her son needed psychiatric help. A family friend, testifying on Shrubsall's behalf at the dangerous offender hearing, told the court that when Shrubsall was a teen, she noticed a large hole he had knocked into a plaster wall in Marge Shrubsall's kitchen. The witness recalled telling Marge that she saw this as a sign that Shrubsall could explode at any time and needed to see a psychiatrist. The woman testified that she then had added, "I know it's shocking, but he could murder you."[17] Marge, she said, "thought about it for a minute and shook her head in disbelief."[18]

The testimony of these women alone, coupled with the crimes for which Shrubsall was convicted might well have been sufficient to convince the Canadian court that the serial rapist was a "dangerous offender" who should be incarcerated for life. But there was much more.

The court also learned that on April 15, 1988, just two months before killing his mother, Shrubsall, then 17, approached a 14-year-old boy at a local bowling alley, grabbed him, kneed him in the head, slammed him against a locker, and then punched him in the face, breaking the boy's nose and leaving him with two black eyes and a swollen lip. At the dangerous offender hearing, this boy, then a young man, testified that he had been playing a video game when Shrubsall attacked him. As if explaining why the boy was about to be assaulted, Shrubsall told him, "You just beat my high score."[19] Although Shrubsall was charged in this attack, the case was referred to the local Dispute Resolution Center for mediation and was resolved out of court by mutual apologies on June 7, 1988, less than two weeks before Shrubsall beat his mother to death.

The sentencing court in Nova Scotia also learned that Shrubsall had harassed and assaulted a number of women between the time of his mother's killing and the crimes for which he was ultimately convicted in Canada. The court, of course, was already aware of the 1995 sexual assault that precipitated Shrubsall's flight from the United States in 1996, but also heard testimony that in 1992, while a student at the University of Pennsylvania, Shrubsall made obscene telephone calls to a female student, who used a telephone company call-back feature to identify him. Questioned at the time about making the calls, Shrubsall did not deny the accusation.

Witnesses also informed the court that, while a student at the Ivy League school in 1994, Shrubsall stalked another woman, a university employee. Shrubsall, the court was told, repeatedly asked the woman out. After several months of being rebuffed, Shrubsall approached her at an automatic teller machine and offered to pay her to give him oral sex. On another occasion, Shrubsall went to the woman's workplace and photographed her. The university responded by providing police protection for the woman.

The Canadian court was also informed that later that year, after Shrubsall had completed his studies at Penn, he volunteered to become an alumni interviewer of students who were applying for admission to the extremely competitive university. One of Shrubsall's alumni interviews took place in the fall of 1994 with a Buffalo area high school senior. Such interviews were generally slated for 30 minutes to an hour and often took place in the alumnus's home. Shrubsall invited this female applicant to his aunt's home in nearby Niagara Falls where he "interviewed" her for four hours, during which he bragged about his accomplishments, belittled other schools in which she was interested, asked inappropriate personal questions, told her she was good-looking and that the University of Pennsylvania needed prettier women, invited her out to dinner, and even kissed her three times. Although this woman rebuffed Shrubsall's advances and decided not to attend the University of Pennsylvania, Shrubsall continued to call her repeatedly for the next 10 months.

Yet another woman told the Canadian court that in 1995 she was taking an evening walk in Niagara Falls when Shrubsall grabbed her buttocks, put his arm around her waist and tried to knock her down. The woman managed to free herself from Shrubsall's grasp and chased him away with a stick until a witness who recognized Shrubsall told her she was "crazy" to be chasing a man who had once killed his mother.[20]

Finally, the court was informed that, prior to the incident in which Shrubsall nearly beat a store clerk to death with a baseball bat, he had been charged with harassing a former girlfriend in Halifax and violating an order of protection she had obtained in an unsuccessful effort to keep Shrubsall away from her. Shrubsall's former girlfriend, whom he had dated for about three months, testified that just five days before the baseball bat attack, she had broken up with him. She told the court that she had seen Shrubsall on the day of the attack, apparently just afterward, as she was headed to court to obtain an order of protection.

Despite the order and her repeated requests to be left alone, Shrubsall continued to contact the woman, barraging her with phone calls, letters, visits, window-peeping and even unauthorized entry into her apartment using a key she was unaware he had. Finally, the local court convicted Shrubsall of criminal harassment, placed him on probation, and ordered him to stay away from the woman for three years. When the harassment continued, the woman went back to court, and Shrubsall was again convicted. Again, Shrubsall was given a break; the court sentenced him to six months of probation and community service.

In addition to all the lay testimony about Shrubsall's violent nature and his harassment of and violence toward women, the sentencing court heard from numerous mental health experts in the "dangerous offender" proceeding.

One was a retired general psychiatrist, whose name was withheld by the court. He testified that he had examined Shrubsall for the prosecution shortly after Shrubsall killed his mother, around the same time that I examined Shrubsall in 1988. This psychiatrist characterized Shrubsall as "bright" but "shifty" and "a bad lot."[21] He added, "As one went on with him, one could see that he wasn't telling the whole truth or that he was varnishing what he did say."[22] The psychiatrist claimed that 13 years earlier, just after the killing, he had diagnosed Shrubsall as a psychopath.[23] If, indeed, this psychiatrist had made such a diagnosis in 1988 rather than 2001, when he testified in the Canadian proceeding with full knowledge of Shrubsall's previous and subsequent history of violent misogyny, it is unclear why this diagnosis was not brought to the attention of the New York courts that sentenced Shrubsall and later granted him youthful offender status based in part on their conclusion that "prospects for defendant's rehabilitation are good" and the fact that the prosecution "did not oppose defendant's request for youthful offender treatment."[24] To put it another way, if this psychiatrist (purportedly hired by the prosecution) had actually made such a diagnosis of Shrubsall in 1988, why would prosecutors and the courts have ignored it?

While there may be doubt as to what diagnoses were made or not made in 1988, there can be little doubt that most of the other psychiatrists and psychologists who testified at Shrubsall's sentencing hearing felt that he suffered from the modern-day version of psychopathy: antisocial personality disorder, which is characterized by "a pervasive pattern of disregard for, and violation of, the rights of others that begins in childhood or early adolescence and continues into adulthood"[25] and is believed by many to be untreatable.

An eminently qualified Canadian team of three forensic psychiatrists and one forensic psychologist testified at the "dangerous offender" hearing. As the court noted, "The experts all arrived at their respective opinions independently. They all made similar diagnoses about the offender's personality without having reviewed each other's reports beforehand."[26]

Curiously, only one of these doctors ever examined Shrubsall. The others relied on a review of records and various psychological checklists in assessing Shrubsall. Interestingly, Dr. Syed Akhtar, the only Canadian mental health expert to actually examine Shrubsall, testified for the defense. Akhtar concluded that Shrubsall was not a psychopath but diagnosed him as suffering from a mixed personality disorder with antisocial and narcissistic traits. Though he did not regard Shrubsall as a sexual sadist, Akhtar concluded that Shrubsall had a "paraphilia" (sexual deviation) characterized by "a predilection for coercive sex with nonconsenting females."[27] He added that Shrubsall showed no remorse, tried to minimize his sexual pathology, and blamed it on his own sexual abuse as a child and the way girlfriends had treated him over the years.

What was the risk of recidivism? And could Shrubsall be treated? The Canadian court summarized the defense expert's answers to those questions as follows:

> Dr. Akhtar was of the opinion that at this stage, it was impossible to say if any treatment would be effective. He noted that treatment of the offender would be difficult and time-consuming because his personality disorder and paraphilia have existed for years. He was unable to say how many years of treatment would be needed to assess its effectiveness. He was, however, able to say that the effectiveness of treatment cannot be judged in a prison setting and whether the offender has modified his behavior will not be known until he is back in the community and exposed to women.
>
> Dr. Akhtar could not say that he saw genuine or enduring motivation. He was skeptical about a number of things the offender told him but especially about his motivation. He noted that the offender could be telling the truth about being motivated yet not have any real motivation. He termed the offender's insight into his problems as dim.
>
> Dr. Akhtar testified that the offender's sense of entitlement (his narcissism) and his antisocial traits make it more difficult for him to control his paraphilia. He could not recall anyone with an antisocial and

> narcissistic personality and paraphilia ever changing. He acknowledged that the success rate in treating persons with the offender's constellation of disorders was not high. He described the offender as being one of the most serious cases he has ever dealt with.
>
> Dr. Akhtar found that, at present, the offender's potential for violent sexual recidivism is high. He pointed out that the offender has never had treatment. He stated that if the offender responds to treatment it is possible that his potential for recidivism will decrease. He noted however that the potential will remain high so long as the offender's attitudes remain the same.
>
> Dr. Akhtar was of the opinion that the offender must be given treatment in order to determine if it is possible for him to change. In other words, to see whether he responds to it. The analogy Dr. Akhtar used was that "you can't win the lottery if you don't buy the ticket."[28]

Given this testimony from his own expert, it came as no surprise to anyone that the court found Shrubsall to be a "dangerous offender" and sentenced him to an indeterminate, possibly life, term in prison. Shrubsall's sentence will be reviewed periodically by the Canadian courts, but he will remain incarcerated until a court determines that he is no longer dangerous to others. Given Shrubsall's history, it will also probably surprise no one if he spends the rest of his life behind bars.

While most would agree that the system finally worked with regard to Shrubsall, many continue to ask why it took so long. Did Shrubsall fool me, the prosecutors, the appeals court, his aunt, and others back in 1988?

To a certain extent, we were all blindsided by the system's failure to record and thus make available to us any record of Shrubsall's troubling and criminal conduct prior to killing his mother. The 14-year-old girl Shrubsall jumped, threatened, and attempted to sodomize in 1986 never reported the incident to the authorities. The two older women who were stalked by Shrubsall when he attended a university basketball camp reported it to the campus police, but that agency apparently handled the matter informally, leaving any disciplinary action to the camp coach's discretion. And the case of the 14-year-old boy Shrubsall assaulted just months before killing his mother was handled outside the criminal justice system, even though under New York criminal law Shrubsall, then 17, was legally an adult.

The psychiatrist purportedly hired by the prosecutors to examine 17-year-old Shrubsall after the killing testified 13 years later that he found Shrubsall to be a psychopath. Today, as then, few mental health experts would countenance placing that label on a juvenile; indeed, the American Psychiatric Association's diagnostic manual, universally recognized as the authority for mental health diagnoses, does not permit a diagnosis of antisocial personality disorder in a person under the age of 18. But if this psychiatrist had so diagnosed Shrubsall in 1988, would the prosecution and the courts have simply deep-sixed his report in a misguided effort to minimize the amount of time Shrubsall spent in prison? Knowing the capable and ethical prosecutors and the "hanging" judge who handled the case, I cannot imagine it.

Perhaps we were all also somewhat blinded by the questions before us. At the guilt-innocence phase of the proceedings against Shrubsall, the prosecutors were not charged with determining whether Shrubsall was dangerous or would harm others in the future. Their ethical duty was to determine what degree of culpability he had for killing his mother and to advocate for what they viewed as a just outcome. They believed, and not without good cause, that Shrubsall was in a state of extreme emotional disturbance when he beat his mother to death. Thus, they fulfilled their professional responsibilities by accepting Shrubsall's guilty plea to the charge of manslaughter rather than murder.

At the sentencing phase of the proceedings, the prosecutors did not contest Shrubsall's request that he be treated as a youthful offender. I do not know why they took that position, but I cannot believe that it was not a principled stance. As far as they and the court knew, Shrubsall had a clean record prior to killing his mother and had great potential that would effectively be destroyed by a lengthy prison term and a lifelong criminal record for manslaughter.

Hangman Hannigan, the judge who denied Shrubsall youthful offender status, was probably the only player in this scenario who actually got the right answer. But even his judgment—which in 20/20 hindsight seems to have been correct—was right for the wrong reasons. He sentenced Shrubsall to 5 to 15 years in prison as an adult, not because he believed Shrubsall was a potential danger to others (at least he never said that was part of his rationale). Instead, Judge Hannigan said he did not believe Shrubsall had been abused by his mother.

Finally, all the players, except Hannigan, relied on my conclusion that Shrubsall had been physically and psychologically abused by his mother and that when he committed the crime, he was, in fact, in a state of extreme emotional disturbance caused by that abuse. I am haunted personally and professionally by what happened in this case: personally because, after decades of working with the victims of violence and sexual abuse, I know all too well the awful harm Shrubsall did to the women he later victimized; professionally because to this day when I testify as an expert, I am often questioned about my role in this case.

As recently as 2005, I was asked in a deposition in an unrelated case whether, after I evaluated Shrubsall, I believed that the killing of his mother was a one-time act of violence for him. Candidly, I responded in the affirmative. Based on the information then available to me, I did believe the homicide was likely to be a single offense and that Shrubsall's prospects for rehabilitation were good. But I also pointed out with equal candor that I did not evaluate Shrubsall's future dangerousness. The question posed to me then as a forensic psychologist was simply, "What was this 17-year-old boy's state of mind when he pummeled his mother to death with a baseball bat?" My conclusion, which I stand by to this day, is that he was in a state of extreme emotional disturbance for which there was a reasonable cause or explanation—the abuse he had suffered that night and for years before at the hands of his mother, abuse that was corroborated by his aunt (his mother's own sister) and other witnesses.

It would be easy to say that I wish I had been charged with evaluating Shrubsall's future dangerousness in 1988, but I would not wish that role on anyone, myself included. Clinical predictions of dangerousness have improved substantially since I examined Shrubsall, but they still rely heavily on evidence of the person's past behavior—the kind of evidence that was available to none of us in the Shrubsall case. Given the state of the art at that time and the hidden record in the matter, I would be the first to admit now that had I attempted to predict the future of 17-year-old Billy Shrubsall, I would likely have failed miserably.

Years later, after Shrubsall fled to Canada and became a brutal rapist, his original attorney, Paul Cleary, responded to claims from some that the system had failed in this case: "It wasn't the system's fault. It was Bill Shrubsall who failed the system. Four judges who never met this kid stuck their necks out for him, showed some compassion, gave him a chance to start a whole new life. He was a brilliant kid. He had great opportunities. He had an Ivy League education. He should be on Wall Street somewhere, making millions of dollars. He threw all that away. Don't blame the system. It's the most disappointing thing I've seen in all my years as a lawyer."[29]

While I agree with part of Cleary's assessment, I also believe that the result in Shrubsall's case was the product of inherent flaws in New York's criminal and juvenile justice systems. In New York, a youngster is an adult for all criminal law purposes at the age of 16. Given the law, which required Shrubsall to be tried as an adult for a crime he committed at age 17, there was no chance that he could be sent to a state youth facility where, over time, his propensity for violence might have been uncovered and treated. The only question left by the law for prosecutors and the courts was how many years Shrubsall would serve in a maximum-security state prison. Given what they knew about him then and the alternatives—a harsh prison sentence that would have destroyed his obvious potential versus a much shorter sentence and expunged record that would only briefly delay his educational and career plans—the decision to opt for leniency made sense.

CHAPTER 7

Battered Woman Syndrome, Duress, and the Death Penalty

7

It was early August 1987 and I was preparing testimony that I would give the following month before a committee of the U.S. House of Representatives, urging Congress to pass legislation giving greater protection to battered women. August has generally been a slow month in my professional and personal life. The university is on summer break, the courts rarely do much business, and the weather in Buffalo is so terrific that there is no reason to leave town. So I had plenty of time to work on my congressional testimony. At least that's what I thought when I answered the phone in my office.

"This is Bob French," the voice on the line announced in a tone that suggested we were old friends, though we had never met or talked before. French explained that he was a lawyer in Fort Payne, Alabama, and needed my assistance immediately: a battered woman was going to be executed unless I said otherwise.

Because I had testified in many cases in which battered women killed their abusers, I had received numerous similar calls over the years; and the volume of the calls had increased substantially in 1987 when my book, *Battered Women Who Kill*, was published. But this one was clearly different. "Did he say *executed*?" I wondered. I had seen many battered women sentenced to life in prison for killing their abusive husbands and boyfriends, but had never heard of one sentenced to death.

French no doubt intended to grab my attention immediately, and he certainly succeeded. I had written extensively about the death penalty, primarily the execution of juveniles and mentally ill offenders but I had yet to work on a death penalty case. I was intrigued by French's bold assertion that I might somehow stop an execution. But before I could get more than a few words in edgewise, the Alabama attorney was off to the races. In about five minutes, I learned the essential outlines of 23-year-old Judith Ann Neelley's predicament.

Judy had been convicted of the heinous torture-murder of a 13-year-old girl and sentenced to die at the age of 18. She was the youngest woman in the United States on death row. French had tried to present a kind of duress defense at Judy's trial, alleging that Judy's husband Alvin had abused her so badly that she felt she had no choice but to follow his orders to kill the child. French had tried to press this defense at trial but was hindered by the lack of an expert witness and was now seeking a new trial for his client based on grounds of newly discovered evidence. The newly discovered evidence of which he spoke was the research that I and many of my colleagues had conducted on the battered woman syndrome in recent years, research that had not been available to French at Judy's trial five years earlier.

French told me that he understood that I was "the world's foremost authority on the battered woman syndrome as a defense in crime" and the perfect person to examine his client, determine whether she suffered from the syndrome at the time of her crime, and figure out whether recent research on the syndrome would have saved her from the death penalty had it been available at her trial and sentencing. That was a tall order, I told French, even for the "world's foremost authority," which, I quickly added, I was not. I named several other experts who might actually qualify for that title and suspected that what French meant was that I was actually the foremost among the authorities who might still be available to him.

There were several "minor" obstacles, I learned. The hearing at which French was hoping to get expert testimony was only a short time away and there were many documents to be reviewed before examining his client. Also, Judy had no funds to pay for an evaluation and the state would pay nothing further for her defense, so both French and any expert he could secure would be working *pro bono* (without a fee). French added that he would personally pay my airfare, drive me from the Atlanta airport to Fort Payne, put me up at his house, and feed me if I agreed to make the trip to Alabama to evaluate his client.

Under the circumstances, I quickly understood why French might be having a hard time finding an expert willing to examine Judy. As I saw it, it was not simply the lack of fee or the timing. The experts I named had all examined and testified on behalf of battered women criminal defendants in the past on a pro bono basis and had not been shy about entering cases at the last minute if that seemed appropriate. Instead, I reckoned that the problem had more to do with the grisly nature of the crime and many experts' reluctance to examine, much less testify on behalf of, an individual who would commit such an awful offense.

None of these aspects of the case troubled me. I was a well-paid professor who could afford to—and felt an obligation to—take on pro bono cases where I could. As it happened, I had the time to tackle the case immediately, so French's short time frame was not daunting. Also, I was not troubled in the least by the nature of the offense. I had evaluated perpetrators of many crimes much worse than those of Judy Neelley. I felt strongly—and still feel—that every defendant is entitled not only to the best defense possible but, where essential to that defense, an evaluation by a competent and independent forensic mental health professional.

What concerned me was whether I could assist French in any way. I explained to the defense attorney that I had examined a number of battered women who claimed that they had been coerced into committing crimes by their abusers, and had even testified in some of their cases. The prognosis for acquittal in these cases, I told him, was grim. Even if I reached an opinion that would support his client's claim, I wondered out loud, whether that opinion would do her any good, especially at this late date when she had already been convicted and sentenced to die. French was realistic about Judy's chances but was a man of amazing optimism, self-confidence, and dedication to his clients. When it became clear that he would not take "no" for an answer, I agreed to review Judy's file and to evaluate her in person. Given the limited amount of time before the hearing, and wanting to minimize trips to and from Alabama, I suggested that I come to Fort Payne and conduct my evaluation immediately before the hearing. If it turned out that I had anything useful to say, I would stay there and testify. If my opinion was not helpful, I'd catch the next flight back home.

I flew from Buffalo to Atlanta and met French, who drove me to the local jail in Fort Payne, about 90 miles west of the airport. I don't know how fast French drove, but I have never covered 90 miles of ground so quickly. I was surprised to find that Judy, who was a death row inmate, had been transferred from state prison back to the small jail in Fort Payne, for a hearing on her petition for a new trial. The jail was old and did not appear very secure. On my arrival, I was greeted by the jail staff, who clearly liked Judy and could not have been kinder and more helpful to me. They escorted me directly to Judy's cell, where I would spend the rest of the day and evening interviewing her. I have examined many dozens, perhaps hundreds of killers over the course of my 30-year career but this was the first and only time I evaluated someone who had already been legally condemned to death.

For someone in Judy's predicament, she was remarkably calm and articulate. She greeted me enthusiastically with the same southern hospitality her jailers had offered me, inquired about my travel, and thanked me for coming. By the time I left her tiny cell many hours later, around midnight and less than 10 hours before the start of her hearing, I had learned a great deal about this young woman and what led her to death row. As a result, I was prepared to testify on her behalf.

Judy was born in Tennessee, one of five children, who lost their father in a motorcycle accident when Judy was nine years old. Thereafter, Judy's mother worked in a factory but had to quit when she became disabled. To support the family, she eventually turned to prostitution. At age 15, Judy met Alvin Neelley, a married man with three children, who was then 25 years old and one of her mother's regular "customers." Judy and Alvin shared a mutual attraction and before long they were lovers. Soon Alvin abandoned his family and ran away with Judy, hoping to establish a new and better life.

But before long, Judy found herself pregnant, working odd jobs, engaging in a variety of crimes, and living in Alvin's car and cheap motels. By the time Judy turned 16, she and Alvin were married and were expecting twins. The twins were born while Judy was serving time in a juvenile facility for armed robbery, and Alvin was imprisoned for his part in the same crime.

Judy was released from juvenile detention in November 1981 at the age of 17. Awaiting Alvin's release, she lived briefly with his parents before she was arrested again for robbery and reincarcerated until March 1982. A month or so later, Alvin was released from prison and the couple reunited and resumed their married life of petty crime, stealing checks and forging money orders. In September 1982, Judy fired a gun into a window at the home of one of her counselors from the youth detention center. A night later, she threw a Molotov cocktail onto the driveway of another counselor from that facility. She then called both counselors and threatened to kill them for abusing her while she was in detention.

Two weeks later, Alvin and Judy kidnapped a 13-year-old girl from a shopping mall. The teenager, Lisa Millican, was with a group of her peers, neglected troubled youngsters from a group home. The couple took Lisa to a motel and kept her there for four days while Alvin beat, raped, and sexually abused her. When Alvin had no further use for the child, he directed Judy to kill her. When Judy's first effort to kill the child—by injecting her three times with a liquid drain cleaner—failed, she ordered her to the edge of a 600-foot canyon, shot her, shoved her over the cliff and watched her body tumble some 80 feet before becoming caught on a tree limb.

During the next few weeks, on at least two occasions, Judy tried unsuccessfully to lure young women into her car. Finally she was able to talk a young couple, Janice Chatman and John Hancock, into riding with her. With Chatman and Hancock in the car, Judy contacted Alvin via CB radio and arranged a rendezvous. Once Alvin joined the group, Hancock said he had to relieve himself. As he walked away from the vehicles down a deserted road, he noticed Judy trailing behind him. He heard Alvin shout that she should hurry up and get it over with. Judy told Hancock to keep walking and then shot him in the back. Hancock fell to the ground and pretended to be dead until Judy left the scene.

Alvin and Judy then took Chatman to a motel where Alvin sexually abused and raped her. A day later, Judy took Chatman into a remote rural area and shot and killed her.

Within days, Alvin and Judy were arrested in Tennessee, the site of the Chatman murder. Alvin tried to blame the crime spree on Judy, telling the police that he and Judy had kidnapped and murdered at least 15 women while working for an interstate prostitution ring, and that Judy was the leader. No evidence was ever found to link the Neelleys to any such alleged crimes.

Alvin led police directly to the body of Janice Chatham and acknowledged his role in her kidnapping and death. Meanwhile, however, he denied raping Lisa Millican and, when police noted that his semen was found in her vagina, he claimed that Judy had masturbated him and used a paper cup to transfer his semen to the 13-year-old's vagina.

Despite his obvious lack of credibility, Alvin was allowed to enter into a plea deal in Tennessee that would spare him any possibility of the death penalty and guarantee him a life sentence. Under the deal he would not stand trial in Alabama for his role in the kidnapping, rape, and murder of Lisa Millican.

Judy was not so fortunate. She was extradited to Alabama to stand trial alone in the kidnapping and horrible murder of the 13-year-old girl. Bob French, who was appointed to represent Judy, agreed to do so for the pittance the state of Alabama allowed the small number of attorneys willing to act as defense counsel in death penalty cases. By the time the case was over, he would have invested thousands of hours and thousands of dollars in the case, making sure that Judy had the best defense he could provide.

French's initial reaction was to consider an insanity defense. It was clear to him that Judy had not been in her right mind when she fell under the influence of Alvin and carried out his orders, no matter how awful they were. But it soon became clear that Judy's involvement in these crimes was not a matter of mental illness but rather coercion. She was not mentally ill in any classic sense of that term, but had been so badly beaten and abused by Alvin that she could not resist his demands—even when they involved kidnapping, assault, torture, and murder.

To prove that, French relied on two witnesses, both of whom had been married to Alvin Neelley. The first witness for the defense was Jo Ann Browning, who had been Mrs. Alvin Neelley for three years before he abandoned her and their three children to elope with Judy. Browning testified that while Alvin had been charming early on in their relationship, he quickly changed into a brutal abuser who beat and raped her almost daily (even during her three pregnancies) and constantly referred to her as a bitch and a whore. On one occasion he punched her in the face and knocked one of her teeth out. At times, he would bite and beat her genitals, telling her that he would make sure that no other man would ever want her. Alvin, she testified, also even tried to rape her 13-year-old sister.

Richard Igou, the prosecutor, belittled Browning's claims of abuse, asking her, "Would you have injected that 13-year-old girl with Drano and Liquid Plumber because you were afraid that he would give you a beating?"[1] After Browning tearfully replied "yes," Igou concluded his cross-examination by asking her four questions, all of which she answered "no": "Did he ever force you to shoot anybody?" "Did he ever force you to pick up a 13-year-old girl?" "Did he ever force you to shoot a 13-year-old girl?" "You don't like Alvin very much, do you?"[2]

Browning was followed to the witness stand by the other Mrs. Alvin Neelley, Judy. One immediate strike against Judy in the minds of those who watched the trial, probably including the jury, was the way she looked. When Judy was arrested, she was a scrawny, dirty, bruised scarecrow of a woman, anything but attractive. Months later when she appeared for trial, she was fashionably dressed, smartly coiffed, delicately made up, and quite good looking.[3] As she stood in court next to Bob French, she looked much more like a young attorney or paralegal helping on the case than a capital murder defendant, a severely abused woman who would claim that she had been beaten into submission and forced by her abuser to commit heinous crimes.

On the witness stand, Judy described how she, too, had initially been charmed by Alvin. Soon, however, she discovered that Alvin's need for sex was insatiable. He demanded sex from her four or five times a day, no matter where they were. Even though she complied with his demands and was with him almost all of the time, he constantly accused her of infidelity. Then the beatings started. Alvin would punch Judy, kick her, and knock her to the ground. Soon the regular routine became a beating followed by forced oral sex. When Judy first became pregnant, Alvin began punching her in the stomach, eventually resulting in miscarriage. Fresh out of the hospital, and still bleeding vaginally, Judy was forced to submit to sexual intercourse. Any resistance on her part was met with even more brutal beatings.

Soon Alvin began raping Judy anally. On one occasion he brutally beat her with the wooden end of a toilet plunger, tried to rip her ears and breasts from her body, and then shoved the plunger handle into her vagina before urinating into her mouth. On other occasions after beating Judy, Alvin raped or sodomized her with a variety of objects, including guns, sticks, and a hacksaw. On one occasion, Alvin forced a baseball bat into her vagina, telling her that that since she "fucked niggers he was going to show [her] how big [her] hole was."[4] French illustrated Judy's testimony by displaying a series of Polaroid photographs Alvin had taken of Judy after he had beaten and raped her. The photos clearly showed many of the injuries Alvin had inflicted, especially those to the most sensitive parts of Judy's anatomy.

Finally, French had Judy explain how the kidnappings and killings came about. Judy testified that Alvin told her that he was "tired of me in bed and wanted me to find him somebody." Alvin, she said, demanded that she pick up girls, bring them to him, and then dispose of them. "He said he was trying to get a virgin," Judy told the jury, "he wanted a tight hole."[5]

After prowling the streets for days, looking for the right target, Alvin and Judy came upon Lisa Millican, who appeared lost. Following orders from Alvin, who was in another vehicle communicating with Judy via CB radio, Judy approached the child and offered her a ride. Lisa accepted the ride and soon found herself in a motel room facing Alvin's demands for sex.

When Lisa refused, Alvin told her that if she continued to refuse, Judy would kill her. Lisa gave in, had sex with Alvin and was raped repeatedly by him over the next several days until, at Alvin's demand, Judy tried to kill the child by injecting her with Liquid Plumber and Drano. When that failed, Alvin became furious with Judy, called her a "bitch," "whore" and "nigger fucker" and threatened to kill her.[6] Finally, Alvin demanded that Judy shoot the child. Judy did as she was told and Alvin stood over Lisa's body and masturbated to ejaculation before Judy shoved the remains over a cliff.

Following the incident, Alvin and Judy went cruising for another "tight hole" for Alvin. Under Alvin's direction, Judy picked up Janice Chatman and John Hancock, and then shot Hancock and left him for dead. Alvin and Judy took Chatman to a motel, where Alvin raped the young woman and then directed Judy to kill her. Again, Judy complied, shooting Chatman twice in the back. Alvin and Judy then went off hunting for another woman to satisfy Alvin's sexual needs. Now, however, Judy could go on no longer. She called and asked her mother to contact the police and have them come and arrest her. Within hours, the kidnapping and killing spree was over.

District Attorney Igou had his work cut out for him. At the very least, he would have to convince the jury that Judy was a victimizer and not a victim. Like most prosecutors cross-examining an allegedly battered woman, he sought to minimize or make light of her injuries. The colloquy went as follows:

Q: How many broken bones did you receive from the beatings?

A: I'll say two fingers.

Q: Never broke your skull.

A: No, sir.

Q: Never broke your arms?

A: No, sir?

Q: Or ribs?

A: No, sir.[7]

Igou then honed in on the two murders, focusing first on the final moments of Janice Chatman's life:

Q: You were afraid somebody would hear her [screaming], weren't you?

A: Yes, sir.

Q: And you shot her twice more in the chest, didn't you?

A: Yes, sir.

Q: Because you were afraid someone would hear her?

A: Yes, sir.

Q: And Al wasn't at your side then, was he?

A: No, sir.

Q: He didn't tell you to shoot her two more times in the chest just to shut her up, did he?

A: No, sir.

Q: You did that on your own, didn't you?

A: Yes, sir.[8]

As for the killing of Lisa Millican, Igou tried a similar cross-examination strategy but didn't get very far:

Q: You injected her again in the neck, didn't you?

A: Yes, sir.

Q: Why did you do that?

A: Because Al told me to.

Q: And you injected her in the arm, why?

A: Because Al told me to.

Q: And you injected her in the other arm, why?

A: Because Al told me to.

Q: And you injected her in the buttock, why?

A: Because Al told me to.

Q: You injected her again in the buttock, why?

A: Because Al told me to.

Q: Did you feel for her?

A: I didn't feel anything.

Q: Actually, what you felt, Mrs. Neelley, was enjoyment, wasn't it?

A: No, sir.

Q: You enjoyed being dominant, didn't you?

A: No, sir.[9]

In an effort to rebut Judy's four days of testimony, Igou called to the stand a psychiatrist, Dr. Alexander Salillas, to testify that, in his opinion, Judy knew right from wrong when she killed Lisa Millican and that she made a conscious decision to do so. On cross-examination, French tried to turn the psychiatrist's testimony to Judy's advantage. French asked Salillas about the concept of "coerced persuasion" and Salillas agreed that "coercive persuasion" can occur "when a husband tells his wife to do something and threatens or intimidates her or beats her into doing it."[10] Salillas also agreed that "coercively persuaded victims usually resist the process initially, but they finally give up."[11] Salillas was helpful to Judy's defense to a point but no matter how hard or long French questioned him, the psychiatrist maintained that people, even battered women, no matter how coerced, always had a choice regarding their behavior.

Finally, French asked if even someone beaten as badly as Judy said she had been would still have a choice to defy her abuser's demands. Salillas replied that if Judy had been beaten as badly as she claimed she "would probably still be in the hospital, would probably be severely damaged all her life, would probably not be so intellectually capacitated to understand [and] probably have every bone broken in her body."[12]

French's cross of the psychiatrist concluded as follows:

Q: And you are on the state of Alabama payroll here today, aren't you?

A: I am working for the state of Alabama.

Q: And you're wanting to cooperate with the district attorney in this case, aren't you?

A: We're after the truth, Mr. French. We're trying to be impartial. You could easily have subpoenaed me to come here, and I would have given you the same answers.

Q: Okay, fine. We'll leave it up to the ladies and gentlemen of the jury.[13]

Following closing arguments, during which French portrayed Judy as a victim of brainwashing and mind control and Igou painted her as a cold-blooded predator, the jury deliberated less than a few hours before convicting Judy of kidnapping and murder. Two-and-a-half hours later, the sentencing hearing commenced and both attorneys renewed their pitches to the jury. Igou, of course, asked for the maximum sentence: death by electrocution. French literally pleaded with the jury to spare Judy's life: "Now I want you to look at this girl because she's a human being. Right now she weeps. Right now she feels, and right now she's so desolate and alone in this crowded room and so helpless. If crying would help, I would cry. If getting on my knees would help, I'd get on my knees. If I could bare my bones for you and save Judy Neelley, I would gladly do it. Don't send this girl to the electric chair. I beg you. I plead with you. Don't do it. Don't kill what God has created."[14]

French's plea worked. In a matter of minutes, the jury reached its decision on sentencing, 10 jurors voting for life in prison and only 2 supporting the death penalty. The jury that heard all the evidence had spoken. That should have been it—and in most states with the death penalty, it would have been. But not Alabama in 1983. The law there at that time gave a single person, the trial judge, the absolute discretion to overrule the jury and impose a sentence of death. And that is exactly what Judge Randall Cole did, announcing that "The court finds by any standard acceptable to civilized society, this crime was heinous, atrocious, and cruel to a degree beyond that which is common to most capital offenses. . . . Accordingly, Mrs. Neelley, the court hereby fixes your punishment at death."[15]

Thus, while a series of plea deals spared Alvin Neelley's life, Judy was sent to death row to await execution. The road from death row to the death chamber is, however, a rather lengthy one in American jurisprudence. Following Judy's conviction and death sentence, French initiated numerous appeals, including a request for a new trial.

It was in his quest to obtain a new trial for Judy that Bob French asked me to evaluate his client and testify at a hearing before Judge Cole. French hoped that my testimony would establish that Judy had been suffering from battered woman syndrome at the time she killed Lisa Millican and that this opinion constituted newly discovered evidence.

Given the history related by Judy directly to me and in her sworn trial testimony, I had no difficulty determining that she was a battered woman who suffered from battered woman syndrome. She demonstrated all the hallmarks of that syndrome as they had come to be known in the eight years or so leading up to my testimony in 1987. In addition to being brutally abused (physically, sexually, and psychologically), Judy had become depressed and hopeless, lost self-esteem, and blamed herself for her predicament, felt trapped in the relationship with Alvin, and had come to feel that nothing she did could prevent the abuse or alter any aspect of her existence.

In my testimony, I explained to Judge Cole the parameters of the battered woman syndrome and how Judy clearly met the criteria for battered woman syndrome as that entity was then understood in the field of psychology. Indeed, I told the court that this was "the most heinous case of wife abuse I had ever experienced or even read about."[16]

I also discussed the very recent understanding of battered woman syndrome and how the term itself was less than a decade old, having been coined in the late 1970s in the seminal works of Dr. Lenore Walker. I added that there had been a "virtual explosion" of research and anecdotal evidence supporting the syndrome within the past half-decade, information that was not available to attorneys such as French at the time Judy Neelley was tried.[17] I was also allowed to describe my own research and that of others regarding myths that both jurors and members of the general public held regarding battered women—that these women remain with their abusers because they are masochists, that they are somehow responsible for and are "asking for" the abuse they suffer, and that they can escape from their abusers by simply leaving them. I told the court that more had been learned about battered women and battered woman syndrome during the preceding four years than at any time in history.

Finally, I testified that, in my view, a battered woman who kills could not get a fair trial unless the jury heard expert testimony regarding the effects of domestic violence and battered woman syndrome because research, my own and that of others, had shown that these concepts were "beyond the ken of a lay member of the jury, in fact beyond that of many in the legal profession."[18]

On cross-examination by an assistant state attorney general, who was part of a special team charged with convincing courts to uphold death sentences in Alabama, I was confronted repeatedly with the difference between Judy Neelley and most battered women who kill: while most battered women who kill take the lives of their abusers, Judy had killed an innocent third party. Under such questioning, I readily acknowledged that this case was unique. The cross-examiner also repeatedly took issue with Judy's accounts of the abuse she said she had suffered, often responding to my descriptions of that abuse by noting

"*If* that's what happened."[19] I could only point to the photographs I had seen, Judy's sworn testimony, and the fact that her description of the abuse and her relationship with Alvin Neelley was consistent with what I knew about battered woman syndrome.

Not unexpectedly, Judge Cole denied Judy a new trial. With regard to the claim of newly discovered evidence, that was supported by my testimony, the judge wrote:

> The petitioner contends that since the time of her trial new research concerning the "battered woman defense" [*sic*] has become available and that such information constitutes newly discovered evidence which entitles her to a new trial.
>
> In support of her claim, the petitioner offers the testimony of Dr. Charles Patrick Ewing, a professor of law and psychology at the State University of New York at Buffalo. Dr. Ewing holds a PhD in psychology from Cornell University and a Juris Doctor from Harvard Law School. He is author of a book, entitled Battered Women Who Kill, and has done extensive research in the field of battered women.
>
> Dr. Ewing testified that the first book on the subject of battered women was published in 1979 and that numerous books and law review articles have been published since that time. He stated that most of the development in that field has been since 1983.
>
> Dr. Ewing testified that research reveals the following about battered women: (1) they are victims of "learned helplessness"; (2) they generally have no community of support because they are frequently isolated by their husbands; (3) the husband demonstrates excessive jealousy manifested by threats that he will kill the wife or their children if the wife leaves him; (4) the wife loses her capacity to make even small decisions; and (5) the husband acquires such control over the woman that she is willing to kill herself rather than kill the spouse.
>
> Dr. Ewing explained that according to a study he has conducted, public opinion stereotypes the battered woman as a person who enjoys beatings, stays with her battering spouse because of some emotional need, and has the freedom to leave him at will, and that because of these stereotypes, it is essential that an accused who is relying on the battered woman defense expert testimony explain the battered woman syndrome.

While Dr. Ewing undoubtedly is one of the country's foremost authorities on the subject of battered women, the court finds that his testimony does not support the petitioner's claim for relief for the following reasons:

1. Although Dr. Ewing concludes that petitioner was a battered woman and acted under the substantial domination of her husband at the time she killed Lisa Ann Millican, he acknowledges that available research shows that when battered women kill, they generally kill their *batterers*. He testified that the case before the court is the only one in which he has been involved where the battered women defense was used to defend against the killing of a person other than the battering spouse. . . .

2. Because none of the studies cited by Dr. Ewing concern homicide or violence committed by a battered woman against persons other than that of the batterer, none of the posttrial developments in the study of the battered woman syndrome, if they had been known at trial, creates a reasonable probability that the outcome of petitioner's trial or sentencing would have been different.

3. Because the battered woman syndrome was developed in 1979, four years before petitioner's trial, evidence of it could have been presented at trial through the exercise of reasonable diligence. . . .

4. The testimony of Dr. Ewing does not establish that the petitioner is innocent of the crime for which she was convicted or should not have received the sentence that she did.[20]

Years later when the case was eventually heard by an Alabama state appeals court, Judy's conviction and sentence would be affirmed but one dissenting judge seemed to agree with French's argument and my conclusion regarding the need for expert testimony at Judy's trial. In an opinion I thought unfairly chastised Bob French, given what he reasonably could have known about battered woman syndrome at the time of the trial, appeals court Judge Fred Steagall wrote:

The most questionable aspect of [French's] strategy was having Neelley testify on her own behalf. French presented no evidence by the testimony of expert witnesses or by other means to establish Neelley's "battered

> wife syndrome" defense, and he never consulted with any mental health professionals to learn about the disorder so that it could be explained rationally to a jury. Instead, French merely had Neelley herself describe her mental condition and her abusive husband. During the four-day direct examination, French elicited damaging testimony about the many lurid aspects of Neelley's life; he also brought out detailed testimony about portions of Neelley's pretrial confession and certain out-of-court statements made by her husband that had already been ruled inadmissible by the trial court and that the State had no way of bringing into evidence. The prejudice that this testimony caused is clear; the trial court's sentencing order shows that it gave weight to her gratuitous testimony when it rejected the jury's recommendation of life without parole and sentenced Neelley to death.[21]

After the Alabama courts repeatedly affirmed Judy's conviction and death sentence over a host of objections, a U.S. Circuit Court of Appeals also affirmed the conviction and sentence, and the U.S. Supreme Court refused to hear the case in 1989, 1995, and 1999.

The Supreme Court's final refusal to hear Judy's case would probably have been the end of the legal road for her. Judy was scheduled to be executed in 1999 and would almost certainly have been executed had it not been for the intervention of the Alabama Governor, Fob James. James had reviewed the entire record of Judy's case, not just her trial, and concluded that she did not deserve to die for her crimes. On January 15, 1999, in one of his last acts in office, Gov. James commuted Judy Neelley's death sentence to life in prison.

While Gov. James refused to give his reason or reasons for commuting Judy's sentence, he later told a reporter, "It would be impossible for me to give you all the reasons without showing you a lot of information and documents on the matter."[22] He added, however, "That DeKalb County jury, which heard all of the facts [of] that heinous crime in the months right after the events took place, convicted her [*sic*] to life in prison. Then, the judge changed the sentence to death."[23]

Subsequently, the Alabama attorney general held that the commutation of Judy's sentence meant that she was eligible for parole. Judy's appellate attorney argued that she was eligible for parole immediately, but a state court held that she would not be eligible for parole until 2014. Even then, she is unlikely to be freed, even if she is paroled. Prosecutors have since vowed publicly that if Judy receives parole in Alabama, they will take every step legally possible to see that she is extradited and tried for the murder of Janice Chatman.

Not surprisingly, in what appeared to be an effort to again reassert some control over Judy, Alvin Neelley responded to Judy's commuted sentencing by telling the press, from his prison cell, that relatives of her victims should "do everything in their power to keep Judy behind bars for the rest of her life, because she's still dangerous."[24] Alvin added that he had been having an affair with Janice Chatman and that Judy "enjoyed shooting her and what it did to me."[25]

There remains debate over whether Judy would or even could be charged with the death of Chatman at this late date. However, should parole ever turn out to be a real option for Judy, she will not have to worry about one thing. Alvin Neelley will have nothing further to say on the matter. On October 21, 2005, he died in prison during surgery at the age of 52.

CHAPTER 8

Validation of Alleged Child Sexual Abuse

8

As a forensic psychologist whose career has spanned over 30 years, it is impossible to forget what can only be described as one of the most shameful episodes in the short history of psychology's influence on the law. In the 1980s, mental health professionals, mostly social workers and unlicensed counselors—but also some psychologists—began a practice known as "validation." These self-proclaimed experts assured attorneys, caseworkers, the police, and the courts that they could simply interview a child suspected of having been sexually abused and determine not only whether the child had been abused but also by whom. From coast to coast, parents who were alleged sex abusers lost custody of their children, while others (primarily daycare providers and preschool teachers) accused of this dastardly offense were sent to prison, not on the basis of any hard evidence but instead on the word of these self-described validators who convinced the legal system that they could divine the truth in these cases.

Child sexual abuse is a scourge that occurs with much greater frequency than many would imagine. The effects of such abuse, though not fully understood, are often devastating. Many cases are never reported because the victims are young, powerless, intimidated, embarrassed, or unable to give a reliable account of their victimization. And, even when child sexual abuse is reported, often little can be done legally because the alleged abuse took place behind closed doors and the only witnesses are the victim and the perpetrator.

Given these characteristics of child sexual abuse, it should come as no surprise to anyone that for decades the legal system has sought ways to more assuredly punish those who engage in such abuse. Protection of our children demands no less. Punishing child sex abusers requires first and foremost a sufficient degree of certainty that the alleged abuser is guilty. In family court proceedings, the burden of proof need be met only by a preponderance of the evidence (more likely than not), but in criminal prosecutions, conviction requires proof beyond a reasonable doubt. That is where the validators came in. They offered the courts something they never had before: purportedly expert testimony that, if accepted by the trier of fact (judge or jury), could easily be viewed as proving by a preponderance of the evidence—and sometimes even beyond a reasonable doubt—that alleged child sexual abuse actually occurred.

The commodity the validators were selling was so desperately desired by the legal system that well-intentioned caseworkers, police officers, prosecutors, and judges were willing to overlook the obvious: it was and to this day remains impossible for anyone, regardless of expertise, training, or experience, to determine whether a child was sexually abused simply by interviewing that child.

But selling phony goods to desperate buyers was only the lesser sin of many validators who developed a cottage industry and quickly became well-paid courtroom fixtures in child sexual abuse cases. A much greater disservice lay in their willingness to find abuse in virtually every case, regardless of the evidence. Countless times, I heard validators testify that if the child said he was abused, that meant he was abused; if the child said he was not abused, that meant he was abused; if the child said he was abused and then recanted, that meant he was abused; and if the child first denied being abused but later changed his mind, that meant he was abused.

My initial reaction to the validators of the 1980s was that they were carried away by greed and a lust for power. I came to realize, however, that while some were so motivated, most were instead good people who felt that they were doing "God's work," so to speak, giving a voice to powerless victims while ensuring punishment for evil perpetrators and protection for potential victims. Many validators must have realized that their "never met an alleged victim who wasn't an actual victim" approach had to result in numerous false positives—innocent defendants who wrongly lost their children or their liberty. But it seemed to me that they saw this as a small price to pay to assure that the vast majority of true perpetrators were punished and prevented from victimizing other children.

My own involvement with the validators came not long after courts first began accepting their testimony. I had spent many years testifying in child abuse cases—both physical and sexual abuse—on behalf of departments of social services and related child protective agencies, and doubted that I would ever find myself on the other side in court. But soon I was receiving frequent calls from defense attorneys asking about this mysterious new process called validation. What these lawyers were describing to me sounded like not just a miscarriage of justice, but a perversion of the principles of psychology.

Soon, I became a frequent witness in validation cases. I never testified that a child was or was not sexually abused. Indeed, in most cases, I was never allowed to examine the child—nor was it necessary for me to do so. My expert testimony in these cases was educational rather than clinical. I took the stand to rebut the often absurd claims made by validators who confidently told the courts that they could determine whether a child had been sexually abused and who did it.

A validator would tell the court that because an alleged child victim demonstrated symptoms such as bedwetting, aggressive acting out, excessive masturbation, or any of a host of about 100 others, this was proof that the child had been molested. I told the court that there was no empirical basis for such claims. Yes, many children who were sexually abused did show some of these symptoms, but so did many more children who had never been sexually abused. There was—and still is—no generally accepted, much less proven, profile of the sexually abused child.

A validator would testify that the behavior of the alleged victim neatly fit what they variously (and often interchangeably) called the intrafamilial sexual abuse syndrome or the child sexual abuse accommodation syndrome. I would tell the court that there was no empirical evidence—indeed no systematic research at all—for these so-called syndromes. Time and time again, I testified that, as any knowledgeable, or even simply objective, observer could plainly see, this emperor had no clothes.

A validator would testify that, because a child kept repeating the same allegations of sexual abuse each time she spoke with a half-dozen or more interviewers or interrogators, the child's account was obviously accurate and reliable. In response, I testified about the growing body of empirical evidence regarding the suggestibility of children, especially very young children.

One validator even went so far as to testify on a number of occasions that children's allegations of sexual abuse were always true because children never lie. Amazingly, in one case, I was called as an expert witness to rebut even that testimony.

Until 1988, all my testimony on the subject of child sexual abuse took place in family court, where the rules of evidence are often relaxed and evidence that would clearly be inadmissible in other courts is frequently accepted by judges (who sit as triers of both law and fact) "for what it may be worth." I was not surprised that family court judges were allowing validation testimony—even before New York's highest court gave such testimony the thumbs-up in family court cases. But I was a bit surprised at the reception my own testimony received from many, if not most, judges. Granted, almost all these judges were from the same county, but I found it hard to believe that they were generally unswayed by—indeed were often hostile to—my testimony pointing out the often obvious flaws in the so-called validations done in these cases.

In retrospect, I realized that my testimony was generally disregarded or given short shrift not because judges did not understand or accept it but because to have given it much credit would have meant rejecting the validation and thus having to tackle the dirty, demanding, and sometimes otherwise impossible job of determining whether the child had actually been abused. Validators, I quickly understood, were so readily accepted by the courts because they made an extraordinarily difficult job relatively easy.

In 1988, I received a call from a public defender who told me that, for the first time in New York, a judge had agreed to allow validation testimony in a *criminal* matter. His client was charged with briefly touching the thigh and genital area of a nine-year-old girl, one of his daughter's playmates, on two separate occasions. After writing a note to her father about the alleged abuse, the girl was interviewed by two police officers, who turned the matter over to the district attorney's office for presentation to a grand jury that heard only the child's allegation and nothing from the alleged abuser.

Although the child told the police she had been touched by the defendant on two occasions about two days apart, the grand jury indicted the defendant on three counts of sexual abuse in the first degree, one for each of three alleged occasions of abuse. Thus, the grand jury must have heard evidence that there were three instances of abuse, as opposed to the two the child had recounted to the police. Given the nature of the allegations, there was no physical evidence.

Prior to trial, the child was interviewed by a validator, the same one who had earlier testified in other cases that children do not lie. This interview occurred 8 1/2 months after the child was interviewed by the police and 10 months after the abuse allegedly occurred. Despite the passage of time, the child gave the validator a much more detailed description of the abuse than she had given the police. Not surprisingly, the validator reached the conclusion that the child had obviously been sexually abused by the defendant—as evidenced by her apparent anxiety and self-reported inability to pay attention at school.

At trial, the judge rejected the public defender's motion to preclude testimony by the validator on the grounds that her testimony would improperly vouch for the child's credibility. The validator was allowed to testify and not only told the jury what the child had said but also gave her own opinion that the abuse had actually occurred, thus implying that the child was telling the truth.

I had no idea whether the child was truthful. My role was simply to explain to the jury that, whatever other evidence there was, the opinion of the so-called validator was not scientifically or clinically reliable.

The result was a battle of the experts, but one in which the prosecution's expert had a decided advantage. She had interviewed the child and told the jury unequivocally that the child had been sexually abused by the defendant. All I could tell the jury was that the validator's methodology was unreliable and explain why. Thus, I was not surprised to learn that, after six hours of deliberation, the jury convicted the defendant on all counts and he was sentenced to 5 1/2 to 11 years in prison.

Naturally, the defendant appealed, and his main claim on appeal was that he had been denied a fair trial by the testimony of the validator who had, in effect, told the jury that the child was truthful in her allegations of child sexual abuse. Testimony vouching for the truthfulness of a complainant is virtually never allowed in criminal cases. As a law professor and criminal law scholar, I believed that the defendant had a valid point. But as one familiar with New York's legal system, I thought it unlikely that the appeals court would agree. I anticipated that the court would find some way to rationalize this gross departure from the normal rules of evidence in criminal trials, given that the defendant had been convicted of molesting a nine-year-old girl.

I was wrong. In a unanimous decision, the appeals court held that the jury's verdict "must be reversed because the court permitted expert testimony of child sexual abuse accommodation syndrome for the purpose of proving that the child was sexually abused."[1]

That landmark decision was rendered in 1990. It is unfortunate that the appeal took as long as it did, for while it was pending, another similar case was tried in an adjacent county. There, too, a validator was allowed to testify against a criminal defendant, but with even more devastating consequences.

In December 1988, 41-year-old Richard Knupp and his 36-year-old wife, Deborah, were charged in Ontario County family court with abusing and neglecting their four daughters, then ages 4, 6, 8, and 10. In November, a school nurse had spotted a bruise on the leg of the oldest girl, who said her father had struck her there with a belt when she refused to take medication for a sore throat. The school's report triggered a child abuse investigation. Before long, without interviewing either parent, the Ontario County Department of Social Services (DSS) removed the children from their parents' custody and placed them in foster care.

While DSS officials did not speak to the Knupps prior to removing and placing the girls, they did obtain information from Deborah Knupp's parents, who had been fighting for almost a decade to obtain custody of the children and later admitted that for years they had been encouraging the girls to tell others that they were being sexually abused by their parents. In fact, Deborah's mother had twice earlier made allegations of child sexual abuse against the Knupps. In 1984, when the family was living in nearby Seneca County, she accused Richard of having oral sex with the couple's oldest daughter but offered to drop the complaint if the Knupps gave her custody of the girl. The Knupps refused and no charges were ever brought against them. When the Knupps moved to North Carolina, the children's grandmother followed the family there and raised the same allegations, which county authorities in that state investigated and found to be without merit.

In 1988, after a limited investigation, the Ontario County DSS alleged that Richard Knupp had beaten all the children with his fist, licked and bitten them all on various parts of their bodies, and placed his finger in the vagina and anus of one of them on many occasions. The DSS also claimed that Deborah Knupp had bitten and struck two of the children, hit one of them with a broom handle, and thrown one of them across the room. The DSS further alleged that the Knupps' home was littered with garbage, spoiled food, open cans, roaches, and other insects; and that the Knupps had deliberately exposed their children to pornographic movies.

The following month, all four Knupp children were examined by a pediatrician. Both younger girls denied that they had ever been touched, kissed or in any way hurt in the area of their breasts, vaginas, or rectums. No clear evidence of sexual abuse was found in the physical examinations of either of these children.

For some reason, the pediatrician interviewed the Knupps' two older children together. Both of these girls told the physician that their father had kissed their breasts but denied any other form of sexual abuse. Based on her physical examinations, the pediatrician concluded that the oldest Knupp daughter's examination was highly suggestive of sexual abuse but not definitively diagnostic of such abuse. The results of the second eldest daughter's physical examination, the doctor concluded, were equivocal.

Both before and after these medical examinations, the Knupp children were interviewed repeatedly by Becky Wendt, an unlicensed counselor who worked for a local rural domestic violence program. At the time of these interviews, according to Wendt, she had "worked with" over 1,000 children, approximately 800 families, and roughly 400 offenders. Her job, she said, was to "do investigative interviewing of [children] to determine their credibility, provide treatment to the child victim and also provide treatment to the offender and the nonoffender parent and any other child in the family situation."[2] The Knupp children, she said, "were referred to me at the end of November by the Department of Social Services due to the allegations of child sexual abuse and I arranged to begin doing a validation with these children to determine if there had been any sexual abuse and, if so, to what extent and by whom the abuse had occurred."[3] Based on her work with the children, she prepared a written report, entitled "The Knupp Validation."[4]

After her validation, Wendt testified before the grand jury that ultimately indicted Richard and Deborah Knupp. Her grand jury testimony cannot be revealed but, after hearing from Wendt and others, the grand jury indicted Richard Knupp on 2,134 counts, including 531 counts of first-degree sodomy, 531 counts of first-degree sexual abuse, 531 counts of incest, and 539 counts of endangering the welfare of a child. The grand jury also issued a 480-count indictment of Deborah Knupp, based on the same evidence.

Although the judge subsequently dismissed the charges against Deborah Knupp for lack of evidence, Richard Knupp was forced to stand trial and three of his daughters testified against him. Based on Wendt's testimony at a pretrial hearing, the girls were allowed to testify via closed-circuit television, outside the presence of their father. Wendt had told the court that "it would be damaging to these children emotionally to testify in front of their father."[5]

The Knupps' oldest daughter, and the only one to give sworn testimony, told the jury that her father "would do this thing called a rib sandwich . . . and he would bite us all over the place."[6] When pressed to say where her father bit the girls, she replied, "Maybe he was just biting them on the arms or like biting them on different parts of the legs."[7] She also testified that her father sometimes "touched" her.[8] Asked where he touched her, she said, "mainly the parts of the legs, parts of the arm or anything like—it's like spots that didn't feel too good."[9] Pressed to be more specific, she replied, "Well, maybe around the private part, but not on it."[10] Pressed further she said, "The back but not the butt."[11] When the prosecutor continued to push her regarding the so-called rib sandwich, she added, "It's not anywhere near the privates."[12]

Asked about watching movies with her parents, she said, "I remember most of them were dirty."[13] Asked what she meant by "dirty," the 10-year-old child replied: "Like ones—like with sexual contact and stuff like monsters and everything."[14] Asked why she watched these dirty movies, she said, "[M]aybe it's because my dad encouraging us to watch them."[15]

Finally, the eldest child testified that her parents had at times "punished" her by striking her with a belt or a broom.[16]

The Knupps' six- and four-year-old daughters testified but not under oath. Under New York law, a child under 10 years old may testify without first swearing to tell the truth but a criminal defendant may not be convicted solely on such unsworn testimony. In unsworn testimony, one of these younger girls, the six-year-old, testified that her father had licked her on her "personals" or "privates."[17]

Becky Wendt, who was also the counselor for all four children, testified at Knupp's trial. Wendt told the jury that her role was to determine the credibility of alleged victims of child sexual abuse and to counsel them if she determined that they were credible. Wendt testified about the five stages of the "intrafamilial child sexual abuse syndrome." Outlining these stages, she told the jury:

> The first step is the engagement stage. This means that a child has, due to being accessible or due to the offender's relationship with them, the offender has an opportunity and control over that child to the point where they are able to—able to begin sexual contact. . . .
>
> When the sexual interaction begins, which is the second stage . . . it begins in a nonsexual manner, where the offender may display some affection to the child or threaten a child, and he gradually begins to fondle the child nonsexually and forces into sexual fondling, mutual masturbation, sodomy and intercourse. . . .
>
> The [next] stage [is] known as the secrecy phase, and that means that in order for the offender to continue contact with that child or continue to have sexual access to the child, he has to make sure that the child is not going to say anything. . . .
>
> The fourth phase is the disclosure phase. . . where a child either accidentally or purposely will disclose sexual abuse. . . .
>
> The last phase is suppression, and this occurs when a child has, following disclosure, the child feels that tremendous sense of guilt . . . because the child feels at that point that they should have either said something before that or other children may have become involved or the offender makes that child feel that he or she is responsible for causing the abuse and for very young children, that feel that, you know, parents are all-knowing and all-seeing; if something is wrong, they have caused this to happen, not—not the adult. . . .
>
> If a child feels a tremendous sense of guilt, several things can happen. They can recant, the can say that the abuse never occurred. Many children will minimize it, they will say maybe it happened once or I can't remember it happening. They will become elective and mute and refuse to talk about it, and some children will self-desecrate, self-mutilate because they are feeling tremendous guilt at this point for what occurred and the disruption that occurred at that time to the family.[18]

Momentarily forgetting that only three of the Knupps' daughters had testified, the prosecutor asked Wendt "In the course of your experience with Heather, Faith—strike that—with Katherine, Faith and

Victoria Knupp, were you able to form any opinion as to the intrafamilial child sexual abuse syndrome?"[19] To which Wendt replied, "I believe the children are certainly very symptomatic of the child abuse syndrome."[20]

The prosecutor tried hard to have Wendt go further in detailing her validation, but even Wendt's statement that one of the girls had told her that her parents "had been hurting her"[21] brought about an objection from defense counsel that was sustained. Since the jury had heard the statement, the judge cautioned the jury: "Mrs. Wendt said that one of the girls or several had said that she was in a foster home because her mother and father had been hurting her. Mr. Cooney [defense counsel] made an objection, I sustained the objection or I have sustained the objection and direct that that statement, had been hurting her, be stricken from the record, and that you disregard that in considering the issues here because it is a hearsay statement, and that is inadmissible before us, so that would be my instruction to you on that point."[22]

Though unable to tell the jury what the girls allegedly told her, Wendt continued her testimony, explaining the basis of her opinion that each of the girls "displayed symptoms common to the intrafamilial child sexual abuse syndrome." For example, as regards the oldest child, Wendt testified:

> [She] initially disclosed information, that sexual information that she felt had been done to her, which was way beyond what a child that age's knowledge and experience. She gave very explicit details concerning when it happened, where it happened, how it happened, what it felt like. She was able to use her senses, touch sense, feel, in terms of what the alleged abuse felt like to her. There was a progression of the abuse over time. She was able to give peripheral details. . . .
>
> [F]ollowing the disclosure, [she] was able to talk to me about this. She felt tremendous guilt over talking about it, feeling something was going to happen to her, this increased over time. She began to become fearful of sleeping. She had nightmares. . . . She felt the alleged offender was going to find her and kill her. Her fears, again, greatly increased until the point she became self-mutilated.[23]

Asked what she meant by "self-mutilated," Wendt explained:

> [H]er eating patterns changed. She couldn't eat or she would make herself vomit. She wanted to punish her body. She felt her body was destroyed by the—what had allegedly happened to her. She, at that point, would refuse to defecate and would constipate herself. She wanted again to punish her organs and again this increased to the point where we felt she needed to be evaluated, due to suicidal ideation.[24]

As regards the six-year-old who testified, Wendt was asked if this child "displayed symptoms of intrafamilial child sexual abuse syndrome."[25] She replied, somewhat cryptically, "Yes. She has been exposed to that"[26] —as though this purported syndrome was a kind of contagious disease. Wendt went on to explain that:

> [The child] gave me information of a sexual nature in which the alleged offenses began with certain types of sexual behavior and increased over time, where she was placed in a position that she allegedly was in the same room with other individuals during the sexual encounters. She also showed very sexualized behavior and was able to talk to me about this. Her knowledge of sexual—sexuality was far above what a child of her age would know. . . .
>
> There were—she alleged that there had been sexual contact between she and another child in the family situation and felt that this was very normal to do. [She] was able to give descriptions of particular events in detail, to give places that this occurred, what happened during those encounters; again, peripheral details that occurred over a long period of time. She was able to tell me what would happen if she told about these alleged incidents. She displayed a great deal of fear that she would be punished or hurt for disclosing to me and, again, as with [her older sister], the nightmares began to increase over time to the point where she was fearful that the alleged person would come into the foster home and find her and hurt her.[27]

Finally with regard to the four-year-old who testified, Wendt told the jury that this child showed "sexualized behavior," reenacted some of the alleged abusive events with "Barbie" dolls, had bad dreams, and sometimes poked herself with a pencil and pinched herself "when she began to talk about the allegations."[28] She added that the girl also "began to have some digestive problems and, again, generalized fears and anxieties over being hurt."[29]

No witnesses were called on Richard Knupp's behalf. But even then, by the time the case went to the jury, the judge dismissed 2,123 of the charges against him for insufficient evidence, leading the jury to ponder just 11 charges. The jury convicted Knupp on all 11 of the remaining charges—sexual abuse and child endangerment—and he was sentenced to 13 to 39 years in prison.

It is likely that the Knupp case would have ended there but for the intervention of Joel Freedman, a local social worker who followed the trial and believed that a gross injustice had been done, and Jack Jones, an investigative reporter for the nearby *Rochester Democrat and Chronicle,* who wrote a series of articles raising serious doubts about the way the case had been handled by the child welfare authorities, the validator, defense counsel, and the court.

Jones pointed out that prosecutors told the court at Knupp's arraignment that he had previously been charged with crimes against his children and that he had previously fled the state to avoid prosecution. Those assertions by the prosecution were used by the judge to impose a bail of $100,000, which effectively kept Knupp locked up prior to his trial. In the face of Jones's investigation, the prosecutor who made those assertions admitted that, in fact, Knupp had never been charged and thus had never fled prosecution.

Jones also learned that the Knupp children's maternal grandmother and her husband had been trying for a decade to take custody of the children from their parents, had previously made a number of unfounded allegations of child sexual abuse against the Knupps, and had encouraged the children to tell people that their parents had abused them.

Jones interviewed a number of close relatives who, despite their dislike for Richard Knupp, asserted that the charges against him were part of a vendetta against Knupp and a plot by the children's maternal grandmother (who had pursued their custody for years) to take them away from Knupp and his wife. These relatives, Jones explained to readers, would gladly have given testimony extremely damaging to the grandmother, and thus to the prosecution's case, but were never called by defense counsel.

Jones further learned that while Knupp had been convicted of child endangerment in part because of the allegations that he showed his daughters pornographic videos, no such videos were found, and video rental records showed that Knupp had never rented any X-rated or pornographic videos. The list of videos he had rented, which included a number of R-rated movies, was found to be inadmissible at trial.

Jones also noted that Knupp's defense lawyer called no witnesses and barely cross-examined the prosecution's witnesses. Jones reported that he had discussed the case with legal experts, who chided the defense attorney, particularly for not presenting expert testimony that would have countered Wendt's testimony.

As for Wendt and her validation testimony, Jones spoke to two local experts, both forensic psychiatrists, who blasted both Wendt and the attorney who defended Knupp.

Each doctor "criticized Wendt for serving as both the children's therapist and as an expert witness for the prosecution."[30] Her dual role in the case, they said, may have contaminated the testimony of the two youngest Knupp girls "by encouraging them to say things they thought their therapist wanted them to say."[31]

Dr. David Barry told Jones that "the only ethical thing" for Wendt to have done was to "decline a request to be the evaluator."[32] Dr. Bruce Kahn, who is also an attorney, said, "The whole question of a therapist being a principal (legal) investigator is very disturbing."[33] Barry added, "This is an important area nationally at this time because of the hysteria that's been introduced into this whole subject of seeking out abuse."[34]

As for the defense attorney's failure to call an expert witness to counter Wendt's testimony, Kahn told the investigative reporter, "That's unconscionable. Expert testimony in a case like this is critical. If the testimony of the prosecution's expert witness was unchallenged, the judge had no choice but to allow it."[35]

Finally, Jones interviewed a number of the jurors who had convicted Knupp. They said they felt they had not gotten the entire story, were shocked to learn that no pornographic or even X-rated movies had been found in the Knupp home, were puzzled that there were "no defense witnesses and no real cross-examination" by defense counsel, and did not feel that Knupp would have been convicted if they had been informed about the background of the children's grandmother.[36]

Editors at the *Democrat and Chronicle* were so impressed by Jones's investigation that they hired an independent, nationally renowned expert to administer a polygraph to Richard Knupp. Warren Holmes, who had previously administered polygraphs for the FBI and the CIA, reported that the results showed that Knupp was truthful and thus falsely accused of sexually abusing his daughters.

Armed not only with Jones's investigations but also Holmes's polygraph conclusions, the *Democrat and Chronicle* published an editorial titled "A Miscarriage of Justice," in which the newspaper's editors charged that Knupp had been wrongly convicted in a trial "studded with irregularities and distortions of fact."[37] The editorial concluded with a plea to the courts to grant Knupp a new trial.

Jones's articles and the paper's editorial caught the attention of many, but none more important than Felix Lapine, a Rochester attorney. Though Lapine had represented criminal defendants for years and had won a reputation as one of New York's premier criminal defense lawyers, I knew him only as a prosecutor. He prosecuted the defendant in the case mentioned earlier, in which the guilty verdict was overturned on appeal because the court permitted a validator's testimony to be used "for the purpose of proving that the child was sexually abused."[38] Though I did not know it when he cross-examined me in that trial, Lapine had been acting as a "special prosecutor" because the local district attorney's office had a conflict of interests that prevented any of its prosecutors from handling the case.

After reading Jones's newspaper articles on the Knupp case, Felix Lapine volunteered to represent Richard Knupp on appeal. Lapine was undoubtedly the perfect attorney to handle Knupp's appeal because he knew from my testimony in the earlier trial that validation testimony was suspect at best and because he had lost the conviction he won in that case because he had presented pretty much the same kind of validation testimony that the prosecutor presented against Richard Knupp.

Lapine appealed Knupp's conviction and while the appeals court held that there had been sufficient evidence to convict Knupp of the charges against him, the five judges on that panel unanimously agreed with Lapine's argument that Wendt's testimony had deprived Knupp of a fair trial. In the words of the court:

> We find the evidence sufficient to sustain defendant's convictions; nevertheless, we conclude that defendant was deprived of a fair trial by the admission of opinion testimony regarding intrafamilial child sexual abuse syndrome. Thus, we reverse defendant's convictions and order a new trial.
>
> Where it is probative, expert evidence concerning rape trauma syndrome and child sexual abuse syndrome is admissible in a criminal case to aid the jury in understanding certain phenomena beyond the common ken. In assessing the probative value of such evidence, the Court of Appeals has recognized "that the reason why the testimony is offered will determine its helpfulness, its relevance and its potential for prejudice."
>
> Here, the opinion testimony was elicited through the People's first witness. After vouching for the credibility of the children, the witness testified about the nature and various stages of intrafamilial child sexual abuse syndrome. The witness further stated that defendant's daughters, who would later testify for the prosecution, exhibited symptoms common to children suffering from intrafamilial child sexual abuse syndrome. In our view, the purpose for which the opinion testimony was offered was to set the stage for the prosecution's case. The witness testified about the symptoms associated with sexually abused child syndrome and then testified that all of defendant's children suffered from those symptoms. Obviously, the prosecution was attempting to raise the inference that, because the children exhibited those symptoms, they had been sexually abused. Where the expert testimony is introduced primarily to prove that a crime took place, its probative value is outweighed by the possibility of undue prejudice.

> Because the testimony was not offered to explain behavior exhibited by the victims that the jury might not have understood . . . we conclude that "such testimony served to bolster the complainants' credibility and interfered with the jurors' duty to assess the complainants' veracity, unfettered and without undue influence by the opinion of an expert." The error in admitting the opinion testimony, under these circumstances, operated to deprive defendant of a fair trial and thus warrants reversal in the interest of justice. Because the People's entire case turned upon the credibility of defendant's children, we conclude that the error cannot be deemed harmless.[39]

Once it became clear that Richard Knupp would be tried again, amazingly the prosecution determined that it would again present validation testimony from Becky Wendt, the expert witness whose testimony caused his conviction to be reversed by the appeals court. I have no idea why the prosecutors decided to use Wendt's testimony in a second trial. Perhaps they realized that their case against Knupp was weak and felt that Wendt's testimony added enough to the case that presenting it was worth risking another reversal. Or maybe the prosecutors felt they could tailor the presentation of Wendt's opinions in a way that an appeals court would not see it as a violation of Knupp's right to a fair trial.

In any event, when defense attorney Lapine learned that Wendt might be testifying in the second trial, he called me; asked me to review Wendt's work on the case, particularly her testimony in the first trial; and possibly testify in the second trial. I was a bit surprised by our renewed contact. As I alluded to earlier, my only previous contact with Lapine had been his cross-examination of me in a case eerily similar to the Knupp case. In that case, he was the attorney who convinced the trial judge to allow a validator to testify in a criminal case.

At Knupp's second trial, only two of his daughters testified and one of them, the oldest, denied ever experiencing or witnessing any sexual abuse. The second oldest Knupp child testified that she had been sexually abused by her father.

Richard Knupp took the witness stand for the first time and admitted that he was an alcoholic who cheated on his wife and brutally beat her in front of their children. He also acknowledged harshly disciplining the children but flatly denied ever sexually abusing any of them. Deborah Knupp testified that her husband had beaten her and that she planned to divorce him but that he had never sexually abused their children. Mrs. Knupp's testimony was echoed in part by that of a number of her relatives, who testified that while they resented Richard Knupp's abuse of his estranged wife, they believed that he was a conscientious father.

Becky Wendt gave an abbreviated version of her testimony from the first trial but maintained her opinion that the Knupp children had been sexually abused by one or both of their parents. But unlike the first trial, this time Wendt was vigorously cross-examined. Lapine focused on her credentials, forcing her to acknowledge that she lacked any formal academic training in the area of child sexual abuse and to concede that at a recent training seminar dealing with validation, she told those in attendance, "we have made a lot of mistakes" in earlier child sexual abuse cases.[40] Lapine responded, "Maybe 20 or 30 guys are rotting in prisons because you made a mistake."[41]

Lapine also confronted Wendt regarding her professional credentials. An unlicensed counselor, she had earlier listed among her professional credentials membership in only one professional organization: the American Professional Society on the Abuse of Children (APSAC). Prior to the trial, Lapine had asked me about membership in this organization as a "credential." I told him that as far as I knew, any professional working in the field of child abuse or some related field could join the organization by filling out a membership application and mailing in a year's dues. A week before the second trial, Lapine, a criminal lawyer with no training and virtually no experience with child abuse issues, was granted membership in APSAC. During cross-examination of Wendt, Lapine showed Wendt a brochure from APSAC and got her to acknowledge that the only requirement for membership was an annual $50 dues payment. Lapine then brandished a document that appeared to be a membership certificate and announced that, like Wendt, he had paid his dues and was a recently minted member of APSAC.

I was called to testify in rebuttal to Wendt's testimony but, according to Joel Freedman (the social worker who had helped Knupp win a new trial), before I testified the prosecutors offered Richard Knupp a plea deal. If he would plead guilty to one of the sodomy charges against him, he would be sentenced to time-served (three-and-a-half years) and would immediately be granted his freedom. Freedman says that Knupp "knew he could face 20 or more years in prison if convicted" but chose instead to take his chances with the jury. According to Freedman:

> He refused the offer because he could not live a lie. Knupp also realized a plea would undermine the integrity of his wife and second [*sic*] child who had testified to his innocence. Knupp was also concerned that a guilty plea would vindicate the system responsible for his unjust treatment and harm others in like circumstances.[42]

Once Lapine had established my credentials, he began his direct examination by having me describe professional standards regarding the assessment of alleged victims of child sexual abuse. In particular, I described the standards of the American Academy of Child and Adolescent Psychiatry (AACAP) regarding the use of anatomically detailed dolls, having one person serve as both therapist and evaluator, and videotaping of the child interviews.

First I testified that contrary to the way they had been used in this case, anatomically detailed dolls were to be used only "sparingly" and "demonstratively"—that is, "where a child is unable to verbalize child sexual abuse, the dolls may be used to help show what happened."[43] Lapine asked me how quickly anatomically detailed dolls had been used with the girls in this case. Although my answer was cut off by an objection from the prosecutor, I believe the jury got the point.

Next I testified that both the guidelines and general position of professionals in the field regarded it as inappropriate for one person to serve as both therapist and evaluator to alleged victims, as had been done in this case. As I explained, in part: "They are roles that are functionally at odds with each other. The role of the evaluator is to determine what happened, find out what happened, and that is often counter-therapeutic to a child. . . . The other reason is that as the child's therapist, you are really being asked to take what the child says at face value . . . in order to help them."[44]

Then, I testified that both AACAP guidelines and generally accepted practice at that time called for interviews with alleged victims of child sexual abuse to be videotaped, something that was not done in this case. Asked why videotaping was encouraged, I explained:

> Well, because unless these sessions with the children are videotaped, we have no way of knowing what really went on. We have no way of knowing what was said by the so-called validator, we have no way of knowing what the child said. . . .
>
> That's one reason. The other reason the Academy recommends, and I think generally people in the field accept it as the standard now, is because it creates a situation where you don't need to have people keep interviewing the child again and again and potentially harming the child.
>
> And then finally the reason is that where there's any doubt in the mind of a court or jury or anybody as to what the child said, you have it right there on tape and it can be shown.[45]

Next, Lapine asked me to address the problems of the kind of repeated questioning of alleged child victims that had occurred in this case. I explained:

> There are two potential problems. One is that the child would be traumatized by repeatedly being questioned again and again about the abuse. That's the danger to the child.
>
> The other danger, a broader danger, is that the child will come to believe things that he or she has said that may or may not be true. Repeated questioning of both children and adults leads them to solidify their memories and leads to very often, especially with younger children, to the point where something may have happened or it may not have happened, but it is impossible to find out because they have been repeatedly questioned about it and the problem is most severe, most serious when the child has been exposed to many questionings and where questions have been used that are leading questions.[46]

Lapine asked me whether, in the documents I had reviewed, I found evidence of leading questions being asked of the Knupp children.

I replied, "Yes."[47] The prosecution's objection was overruled, and Lapine than asked, "What else, if anything, is the appropriate way to go about questioning children about accusations such as have been made here?"[48] I replied, tacitly criticizing what had been done in the evaluation of the Knupp children:

> First of all, you have to do a thorough evaluation of the child. You have to do, not only an evaluation of what the child said happened, but a thorough psychological evaluation of the child.
>
> You have to know what the child's intellectual functioning is, cognitive functioning is, emotional and social functioning are. You have to interview the parents, you have to get the detailed developmental history.
>
> It's not something that you can accomplish just by talking to the child himself or herself.[49]

Lapine responded by asking, "In this case what was done?" But before I could reply, the prosecutor objected.[50] Although the judge overruled the objection, saying "I assume that we are talking about what Mrs. Wendt testified to here today," Lapine moved on to another topic, apparently satisfied that the jury understood the significance of what I had said.[51]

On cross-examination, the prosecutor spent little time on the facts of the case, instead emphasizing my training as a lawyer as well as a psychologist, my compensation, and how many times I had testified for prosecutors as opposed to defense attorneys. She also spent some time trying to paint my testimony regarding videotaping and dual roles (therapist-evaluator) as simply my own opinions. I agreed with her assertion that some people might well disagree with me.

Then the prosecutor resorted to a ploy often used in cross-examining an expert witness. She got me to readily agree that Dr. Lenore Walker, an esteemed colleague who coined the term "battered woman syndrome" was an expert on that subject. Then the prosecutor asked: "And if I were to tell you that Lenore Walker has stated in an interview that there are times when it is perfectly appropriate to provide treatment for—and testify in court on behalf of abused children, would you disagree with that?"[52] Felix Lapine's objection to the question was sustained by the judge before I could answer. Thereafter, much of the remaining cross-examination devolved into what even the judge acknowledged was an arguably irrelevant discussion of battered woman syndrome. It appeared to me that the prosecutor was trying to make a psychological connection between battered women and sexually abused children—a connection I accepted as generally valid.

Two days after I testified as the last witness for the defense, the jury acquitted Richard Knupp on all 11 remaining charges, and he was freed from custody for the first time in over three-and-a-half years. His freedom was, however, stressful and short-lived. His wife followed through on her stated plan to divorce him, a family court restraining order prevented him from seeing his children, and five-and-a-half years after his acquittal, he died of colon cancer at the age of 49.

CHAPTER 9

Murder or Manslaughter? Extreme Emotional Disturbance

9

By age 29, Rudy Manzella had fallen into a predictable lifestyle. Most people his age would not have been satisfied with the life he was living, but to Rudy the dull routine of his existence was both manageable and comfortable.

Having dropped out of school in the ninth grade and never married, or even had a girlfriend, Rudy had spent his whole life living in Clarence, New York, then a rural area outside Buffalo, with his parents. He drove a car for awhile when he was younger but, after two arrests for driving while intoxicated, had given it up and found it easier to get around on foot or on a bicycle. He tried working but couldn't hold a job because he could never seem to work fast enough. Eventually, he found a job he could manage. For five or six years, he had been employed at a nearby pizzeria, where his job was to assemble folded pizza boxes. He was a good worker, enjoyed the challenge of this seemingly mindless job, and often went to work a couple hours early and even on his scheduled days off.

When Rudy wasn't working, he mostly stayed at home, drinking beer; watching cartoons, wrestling, and videos; and caring for his dogs.

Other than going to work or to the store, Rudy's forays into the community were pretty much limited to visiting family. On May 27, 1989, Rudy spent the night at the home of one of his younger brothers in Tonawanda, another Buffalo suburb. The next day, when Rudy awoke, he was hung over, so he called his boss to say that he couldn't make it to work that day. The boss refused to give Rudy the day off and when Rudy objected, he was fired. Losing his job spelled trouble for Rudy, but was only the beginning of the turmoil that was about to consume his life.

Hours after being told that he was fired, Rudy argued with his brother. His brother responded by ordering Rudy to leave. It was dark outside when Rudy left his brother's apartment and began what would have been a good 15- to 20-mile walk home. Before long, he was stopped by a police officer and asked where he was going. The officer was likely taken aback by—if not suspicious of—Rudy's explanation that he was walking home, given the great distance he would have had to cover on foot to get there.

When the officer tried to question Rudy, he took off running back toward his brother's apartment. The police officer chased Rudy down and saw him throw a straw to the ground. As it turned out, the straw appeared to contain residue of cocaine, so Rudy was taken to the local police station and released with an appearance ticket—essentially a warrant requiring his appearance in court on a later date.

Seventeen days later, Rudy returned to court in Tonawanda as required by the ticket. The court was located in the same building as the town's police headquarters. Rudy waited for his case to be called, pleaded not guilty, was told by the judge that he could obtain a lawyer from the assigned counsel program, and was taken from the courtroom by police officers to be fingerprinted.

Before Rudy was fingerprinted, two of the officers asked him if he liked boys. One of the officers told him, "You look like a faggot, probably like little boys."[1] The officers then repeated these taunts and began fingerprinting him. One officer told him, "If you don't get it right, I will stick you in a cell back there, and I might not get it done until tomorrow."[2] As Rudy was trying to cooperate with the fingerprinting process, he found himself standing behind one of the officers. Another officer said to Rudy, "What are you trying to do, butt-fuck him, make love to him like a faggot or something?"[3]

One of the officers then asked Rudy if he wanted to make a deal. Rudy told the officers, "I'm not blowing anybody in," meaning he would not tell them the source of any drugs he may have possessed.[4] The officer replied with an accusation that Rudy had raped two young girls. The officer told him that the police had a picture of him, "positive identification."[5] They added, "People said they saw you rape a seven-year-old and an 11-year-old and made them give you a blow job on Fletcher Street."[6] The officers told Rudy they knew he was the alleged rapist, the cocaine charge was "nothing," and that they would have him locked up for life in prison where he would "get all the sex you want."[7] One of them added, "You're not going to get a lawyer."[8]

Rudy asked about the lawyer the judge said he was entitled to, but one of the officers told him that the judge had lied and that Rudy could not see a lawyer. Rudy then asked to see the picture that supposedly had been used to identify him as a child-rapist. One of the officers, a detective, responded by grabbing him, knocking him down into a chair, telling him to be polite, and then adding "If I see you in this town or building, I will throw your ass in jail. Don't ever come back."[9]

Upset and frightened, Rudy fled the building. He stopped at a supermarket, bought a beer, and ran to his brother's apartment. His brother then drove him to his parents' home in Clarence. During that trip, Rudy slumped down in the car, trying to keep from being seen by the police.

When Rudy arrived at his parents' home, he appeared to be terrified. He told members of his family that he was afraid that the Tonawanda police were going to frame him for raping a child and send him to prison, where he would be locked up for life and beaten and raped until he died. Over time, he expressed these fears repeatedly along with his conclusion that the only way to avoid such a fate was "just not to go back, never go back to Tonawanda."[10]

Though he had no intention of ever returning to the court in Tonawanda, Rudy did make some efforts to get an assigned attorney. Since no public defenders served the court in which he was charged,

Rudy had no choice but to call the local assigned counsel program. Under their rules, to qualify for an attorney, he first had to establish his inability to pay for private counsel. In his numerous telephone contacts with the assigned counsel program, their staff quizzed him regarding whether he had quit his job or been fired, whether he was getting unemployment benefits and, if so, how much money he was receiving. Rudy felt that he was being put through needless "red tape," which may or may not have been the case. In any event, given that he had been told flatly by the police "You're not going to get a lawyer," it seems quite understandable that after several fruitless phone calls and a letter, Rudy gave up on getting an assigned attorney.[11]

Terrified at the thought of returning to the Tonawanda court, and having no access to counsel, Rudy adopted a strategy of denial. He repeatedly told family members that he would not return to Tonawanda to face the charge against him and that if the police tried to force the issue they would have to kill him or be killed. Obsessed with the idea that the police might come for him at any moment and that he would have to protect himself from arrest, he began drinking heavily, sleeping with a gun beside his bed, and ignoring demands that he return to court.

Rudy's strategy seemed to work, at least until October 20, 1989. On that morning he was awakened by his brother who told him that he had a phone call from a Tonawanda police officer who had a warrant for his arrest. Rudy took the phone and spoke to the officer who explained that Rudy had to appear in court that day but could be bailed or possibly even released with just a fine. Rudy, who believed that the officer was toying with him and getting "some kind of sexual thrills from tormenting" him on the phone, told the officer, "Fine, just don't come over here." To which the officer replied, "I will do what I have to do."[12]

At that point, Rudy believed that the Tonawanda police might actually be coming for him. He showered, dressed and went to a nearby store to buy a quart of beer. Rudy then settled before the television set to watch *Beverly Hills Cop II*. Beside him, he had a loaded rifle. Sitting there, expecting the police to show up at any time, he thought, "If they came to get me, they would lock me up for life. I was going up for rape.

Nobody could help me or even find me. . . . I thought I was going to die in jail, I might just as well die at home."[13]

Suddenly Rudy's ruminations were interrupted by the sound of his dog barking. Rudy ran to the kitchen window and saw two marked squad cars, which he assumed were from the Tonawanda Police Department. In fact, the two cars were county sheriff's vehicles. The Tonawanda police had asked the sheriff's office to bring Rudy in.

Seeing the police cruisers, Rudy grabbed his rifle, aimed it at one officer through the glass window, pulled the trigger, and saw that officer fall to the ground. Rudy then watched as the other officer got out of his vehicle and reached for his gun. In response, Rudy turned the gun on the second officer and shot him three times.

Rudy's plan at that point was to shoot himself, but he never did so. Instead, other police officers responded to the shootings almost immediately. One of the wounded officers was dead on arrival at a nearby hospital; the other was critically injured but would survive. Police surrounded the Manzella residence, setting into motion what would turn out to be an eight-hour siege, much of which was captured on tape as police officers used telephone calls to try to talk Rudy into giving himself up.

During the course of these conversations, Rudy (who had been told that neither of the officers he shot was dead) made several references to the earlier misconduct of the Tonawanda police. For example, at one point early in a recorded conversation with Officer Dennis Rankin, the dialogue went as follows:

Rudy: I'm saying there's crooked cops and why—why—where the hell am I going to get (unintelligible). I went to court last time and listened to (unintelligible) kind of bullshit and I got beat up.

Rankin: I know that.

Rudy: The guy says don't come back. I don't come back and now I got a warrant for my arrest again. How much fuckin' money you think I got? I don't even got a job this month.

Rankin: [I]f you're not worried about Rudy, for Pete's sake, worry about your Mom. Okay? Mothers are forever, Rudy, mothers are forever.

Rudy: (Unintelligible) Mom. Alright, let me explain this. I'm worried about her. What do you want me to do?

Rankin: I want you to come out and ta—

Rudy: Want me to go to jail for the rest of my life for her? Five years, 10 years, get beat up from all the faggots? What do you want me to do, get accused of rape while I'm there. What can I do in there, staying for the rest of my life. If I'm only sentenced to five years. What other fuckin [*sic*] law can I get broke in there, that I can break. . . . I mean like what else can you set me up for. What do I look like a fuckin [*sic*] idiot or can you get your shit straight this time.[14]

Ultimately, the standoff ended peacefully when Rudy surrendered to the police and was charged with multiple crimes, including the murder and attempted murder of a police officer.

Rudy, who was unable to get a lawyer to represent him on the misdemeanor drug charge in Tonawanda would soon be represented by one of New York's top criminal defense attorneys, Joel Daniels. Faced with a client who had killed one police officer and grievously wounded another, Daniels had little choice but to consider a possible psychological defense, either insanity or extreme emotional disturbance. Within two weeks of Rudy's arrest, he contacted me and asked me to evaluate his client. Over the next six months, I would examine Rudy on five occasions and conduct psychological testing with him on two of those occasions. I would also listen to the telephone tapes of his standoff with the police, interview his relatives, and review thousands of pages of records.

Because Rudy had shot and killed a police officer, there would be no plea bargaining. He could either plead guilty and face 50 years to life in prison or go to trial and, if convicted, face the same sentence. Thus, he had nothing to lose by going to trial, whether he had a defense or not. As it turned out, however, after six months of intensely studying Rudy and his crimes, I reached the conclusion that he was in a state of extreme emotional disturbance at the time of the shootings. Thus, Rudy would have not only a trial but a defense.

A year later, in June 1991, when a jury finally heard the case, it was clear that the trial would be the classic battle of the experts. I would testify for the defense and the prosecution would call Russell Barton, MBBS, who had earlier testified in the John Justice case, and Dr. Morris Newman, a local clinical psychologist. On the one hand, I was quite familiar with Barton, and there was no mystery as to what his testimony would be, even though I had never seen a report from him. Newman, on the other hand, was harder to predict. I had never met the man or even heard of him. As far as I knew, he had not testified before. Newman had done psychological testing with Rudy, and his report generally supported the conclusion that Rudy was emotionally disturbed at the time of the shootings. Thus, as I took the witness stand, I was unsure whether Newman would even be called as a witness.

My direct testimony was designed to tell the jury my opinion and to explain it. But Daniels also used my testimony as an occasion to get Dr. Newman's findings before the jury in the event the prosecution chose not to call him as a witness. As an expert witness, I was allowed to describe to the jury any evidence I relied on in forming my opinion. In this case, although I felt it was somewhat flawed, Newman's testing was certainly one piece of evidence on which I had relied.

In my view, Rudy was a troubled young man whose psychological development had essentially ceased when he was in his early teens. As I explained to the jury:

> His mother described him early on as a fast learner. As an infant, [he] walked early, talked early, didn't attend preschool, was eager to attend kindergarten, did very well in kindergarten, enjoyed school and adjusted well to elementary school. And generally did well in life until around the age of 12 at which time he started to have trouble at school, started running away from home. In his Mom's words, "Went from being a sweet kid to a little snot you wanted to smack." Junior high school the

> problems continued and his family members described him as stopping developing at that time. Finally his mother gave in to his demands or requests that she sign for him to quit school. He did quit school before finishing. His adulthood, that is his chronological adulthood. The years thereafter he never left home, was content to live at home. Basically worked, watched t.v., drank beer, had no relationships outside the family, never dated. His family regarded him as funny and treated him kind of like a family pet. He was never dependable, always dependent on others, took 30, 45 minutes to do any task, even the simplest task that he was asked to do. His only real work experience in life was folding boxes at a pizza restaurant called Pizza Junction. He enjoyed folding boxes and did a good job there, and enjoyed doing it so much he would go in several times early on his own time without pay, folding boxes.
>
> . . . He never developed adult interests, never had a social life outside the home, spent time as an adult living at home, never left home, watched cartoons every day, taped them, watched the same ones over and over again, seemed to live in a fantasy world, believed that wrestling and martial arts movies were real, and one of his brothers told me that he even believed that some cartoons were real. He would go around the house acting out scenes from movies singing songs. He went through a period of [a] number of years as a person in his middle twenties pretending that he was Elvis Presley, acting like Elvis, combing his hair like Elvis.[15]

Daniels asked if I could say what had caused Rudy's obviously abnormal behavior and I replied: "I don't think anyone knows. I can't tell you with any degree of certainty why he stopped developing. All I can tell you, in my estimation, he functions at around age 10 to 12 range. He just really never went beyond that. His development was arrested."[16]

Next, I testified that I had given Rudy an intelligence test, the Wechsler Adult Intelligence Scale, on which he had achieved a full-scale IQ of 82. I further explained that while the diagnosis of mental retardation was not warranted in Rudy's case, under the *Diagnostic and Statistical Manual of Mental Disorders* (Third Edition, Revised), which was then the prevailing standard, an IQ in the range of 71 to 84 was considered indicative of borderline intellectual functioning.

The questioning turned next to Dr. Newman's testing of Rudy. Newman had given Rudy the Wechsler Adult Intelligence Scale just four days after I had administered the same test. By Newman's calculation, Rudy had a full-scale IQ of 91. It was never clear to me why the psychologist had given Rudy the same test less than a week after he had already taken it. However, it seemed clear to me—and I testified—that this was not proper practice and that Rudy's score on the second administration of the test was likely inflated by what psychologists refer to as practice effects. As one authority has recently described them: "*Practice effects* refer to gains in scores on cognitive tests that occur when a person is retested on the same instrument, or tested more than once on very similar ones. These gains are due to the experience of having taken the test previously; they occur without the examinee being given specific or general feedback on test items, and they do not reflect growth or other improvement on the skills being assessed."[17]

In my experience, to which I also testified, Newman should have waited approximately six months before giving Rudy the same intelligence test in order to avoid the taint of practice effects.

Interestingly, and again surprisingly, on May 17, 1990, Newman had given Rudy the Minnesota Multiphasic Personality Inventory (another widely used psychological test known as the MMPI-2). I had given Rudy the same test on March 20, 1990, less than two months earlier. There seems to be less agreement among experts regarding the problem of practice effects on the MMPI-2, but readministering it within such a short time span certainly raised questions about its usefulness.

My interpretation of Rudy's MMPI-2 profile, to which I testified, was:

> In summary fashion, what it shows is an individual who was in a great deal of psychological turmoil, who was immature, dependent, anxious, tense, nervous, depressed, apathetic, pessimistic. Someone who has unusual and unconventional ideas about his environment. Someone who obsesses or thinks about things over and over again, and who probably suffers from delusional thinking at times. And overall, it's consistent with someone who has serious mental problems.[18]

Asked to relate to the jury Dr. Newman's conclusions from Rudy's MMPI-2, I testified that according to Newman's report, Rudy was likely to exhibit a thought disorder, that his thinking was "fragmented, autistic, tangential" and marked by "paranoid features."[19] Allowed by the court to refer directly to Newman's report, I read the jury the following conclusion: "The prognosis is generally poor. The problems of these individuals most often are chronic and severe, although their ability to work may not be severely impaired."[20] As for diagnoses, I also told the jury that Newman's report called for the need to "rule out" (give further consideration to) organic disorders, paranoid schizophrenia, paranoid disorders, and schizoid personality disorder.[21]

Before getting to my ultimate opinion regarding extreme emotional disturbance and the bases for that opinion, Daniels asked how, if at all, I corroborated what Rudy had told me and his family about how he had been roughed up and threatened by the Tonawanda police. First, I explained that "[T]he testing indicates that this is a very simple-minded individual who, basically, what you see is what you get. There is very little ability to fake or to concoct a lengthy scenario of this nature."[22] Then I turned to videotapes I had reviewed showing the behavior of the detective Rudy claimed shoved him down, threatened him, and told him never to come back to Tonawanda.

As I testified, the first of these videotapes showed that detective assaulting a man who was charged with drunk driving and being booked at the Tonawanda police station. Asked how, if at all, I found this tape corroborative of Rudy's description of being abused by the police, I explained that the video "showed the capacity of the individual he said abused him for this kind of abusive behavior to suspects."[23]

As for the second videotape I reviewed, I testified that it showed a local television reporter trying to interview the same detective. Although the prosecutor objected to my describing what I saw on that videotape, the judge allowed me to testify how what I saw there corroborated Rudy's complaints about this detective. The detective's response to the reporter, I told the jury, was "consistent with the kind of abuse that Rudy Manzella described to me."[24]

In concluding my direct testimony I reiterated the reasons for my opinion that Rudy had been in a state of extreme emotional disturbance when he shot the two police officers who had come to arrest him: his limited intellect, his immaturity, his long-standing emotional problems, the way he had been treated earlier by the Tonawanda officers, the absolute dread of going to prison inspired by those officers, and his state of mind as revealed in the telephone tapes of the eight-hour standoff with the police.

Cross-examination was conducted by prosecutor George Quinlan, who had earlier cross-examined me in the John Justice trial, so I knew much of what to expect. As anticipated, there was the obligatory line of questions to establish that as a psychologist I could not perform surgery, prescribe medications, or conduct medical tests such as X-rays. Also as anticipated, Quinlan noted that I hadn't ever testified at trial for his office (the Erie County District Attorney), brought up my testimony in the Judy Neelley case in Alabama, and attempted to paint me as a psychotherapist who tried to talk people out of their mental problems.

The prosecutor also threw in a few new items I hadn't expected. He established that as a psychologist, I could not give an opinion to a reasonable degree of *medical* certainty, rather to a reasonable degree of professional certainty or scientific certainty. He also asked me to acknowledge that battered woman syndrome—a topic about which I had written and testified extensively but which had no bearing whatsoever on Rudy's defense—was not a diagnosis found in the *Diagnostic and Statistical Manual of Mental Disorders* (Third Edition, Revised), also known as the *DSM-III-R*. That question and my response were followed by what I can only describe as the strangest line of courtroom questioning I have ever undergone, seen, or even read about:

Q: And we have already established, I guess recognized the *DSM-III-R* as an authoritative reference?

A: Yes.

Q: That publication contains a listing of accepted mental disorders in this country?

A: Yes.

Q: It's published by a—the American Psychiatric Association, correct?

A: Right.

Q: And your copy [is] the paperback version of the hard-bound copy I have in my hands?

A: Right.

Q: That's the one with the figure, the sketch of Benjamin Rush?

A: Yes.

Q: You know who he was?

A: Yes. Father of American psychiatry.

Q: His claim to fame was that, among other things, was that he signed the Declaration of Independence.

A: I don't know that was his claim to fame. He did sign the Declaration of Independence.

Q: Perhaps you're more familiar that he thought mental illness was caused by bad blood in the head. To treat the illness he would bleed the veins in people's heads.

A: I'm not familiar with that.

Q: That's the guy they continued to use as a logo for their book.

A: Whatever he did, he is recognized as the father of American psychiatry. He is not my father.

Q: I am not suggesting that he is.

A: No, but I don't have any particular regard for him, whatever. I don't get your point. I don't get the point about Benjamin Rush.

Q: Let's move on.

A: Yes.[25]

While I found this line of questioning bizarre to say the least, what caught me most by surprise was something I probably should have expected: Quinlan's effort to get me to help him undermine the findings of his own expert, Dr. Newman—findings that were helpful to the defendant's claim of extreme emotional disturbance.

After establishing that MMPI-2 profiles are often scored by computer and that both mine and that of Dr. Newman were so scored, we got into the distinction between psychologists who, like me, rely on computers simply for raw scoring and others who rely on a computer program not only to score but to interpret the MMPI-2. Dr. Newman had produced an MMPI-2 report in this case that was generated by an interpretive computer program. I do not rely on such programs because, when cross-examined, I cannot explain to the questioning attorney how such programs work since the algorithms they utilize are generally proprietary and not available to me.

The prosecutor was angling to diminish if not destroy the value of the MMPI-2 profile generated by or for Dr. Newman in this case:

Q: You punch in all the answers there, run off the computer, you come up with something like Dr. Newman did.

A: Right.

Q: Really, all this is, those items that you referred to testifying on direct about Dr. Newman's report, all that is, is a printout which is generated by some people who said, if you get certain answers to certain questions here is what you should be looking at, right?

A: Yes, pretty much. It's his report, however, he put his name on it; he stands behind it.[26]

After establishing that Dr. Newman's MMPI-2 interpretation was probably generated by a computer program prepared by the staff of Psychological Assessment Resources, Quinlan tried—in my view, unsuccessfully—to further distance Newman from the conclusions in his report:

Q: They made the software, but the language contained within the interpretative report is the language of Roger Green, Robert Brown and the PAR staff?

A: That I couldn't tell you. I don't know. All I know is that it says Morris Newman, PhD, on it.

Q: Right to the left of where it says Morris Newman, PhD, it says prepared for Morris Newman, that's what you know?

A: Right.[27]

After establishing that I had completed my own interpretation of Rudy's MMPI-2 profile, Quinlan asked me to compare mine with Newman's computer-generated interpretation. "Which one is more accurate, yours or his," he asked.[28] "I think they're both accurate," I replied.[29]

The prosecutor then turned back to Newman's computer-generated report and might have scored a few points had he not pushed his questioning as far as he did:

Q: [Pointing to Newman's computer-generated report] And what it says there that this is an—the interpretation contained in this report should be viewed only—or excuse me should be viewed as only one source of hypotheses about the individual being evaluated. What's a hypothesis?

A: Typically, a hypothesis means a theory, well defined, well specified theory that is testable.

Q: So when this scoring service sends back a report like this, they're not saying this is the gospel truth? They're saying here is a hypothesis based upon the answers the subject gave to your test, right?

A: Right.

Q: And like in any hypothesis or theory it can be tested and found out to be true, correct?

A: Yes.[30]

Defense attorney Joel Daniels realized what was happening in this line of questioning and rose to object, telling the judge, "Your honor, I object to the characterization [']hypothesis[']. Mr. Quinlan, for some reason, is knocking his own psychologist's report. That's his business. He is plainly trying to characterize what is plainly written in the interpretative portion of that report as a hypothesis. That is not true."[31]

Quinlan ignored the objection—as did the judge, apparently—and kept on questioning me, finally pointing to the computer-generated MMPI-2 profile and saying: "This is no different if someone sent in one of these astrological charts."[32] Obviously I disagreed with that characterization.

Quinlan may or may not have made his point but, in any event, would not let it go until the judge stepped in and forced his hand:

Q: [Pointing to Newman's MMPI-2 report] You are citing the report of Dr. Green and Dr. Brown?

A: No. Dr. Newman's report.

Q: This report was prepared by Dr.—

A: We can quibble over the words. He submitted it to you, did he not?

Q: Let me see if we have the same document.

The Court: Let's not quibble. If that report was submitted by Dr. Newman under his name, it's his report.

Mr. Quinlan: It is indicated that it was prepared for Newman.

The Court: Newman accepted it and submitted it, so let's not quibble; and I think that these questions and these answers are starting to get beyond the ken of this jury. Let's start—

Mr. Quinlan: I just have a couple more.

Mr. Daniels: It should be made clear that those reports were submitted on behalf of Dr. Newman, the Prosecution's psychologist in this case.

The Court: If Newman got a report from the moon and put his name on it, it's his report.

Mr. Quinlan: Prepared for Dr. Newman by somebody on the other side of the moon.

The Court: If he accepts it, puts his name on it, it's his report.

Mr. Daniels: They can't have their cake and eat it. He was their psychologist.[33]

Regardless of the effect this line of questioning may have had on the jury, Quinlan also struggled to undermine my conclusion that Rudy's functioning was more like that of a 12-year-old than a 31-year-old and my belief that Rudy had actually been abused by the Tonawanda police:

Q: Now, how many people who are 31 years old have you seen who act like a 12-year-old?

A: Not very many.

Q: So are you experienced with those kinds of people?

A: I am very experienced with 12-year-olds. I have examined dozens, perhaps hundreds.

Q: Let's talk about somebody who is 30 years old, when you first saw the defendant, right?

A: Right.

Q: So you are saying he lived and acted like a 12-year-old?

A: In many ways, yes.

Q: Did he drive an automobile?

A: Not for a number of years after he lost his license.

Q: Do 12-year-olds drive automobiles?

A: Some do. Most don't.

Q: He drove an automobile as an adult, right?

A: Right.

Q: Drank alcohol as an adult?

A: Yes.

Q: 12-year-olds don't drink alcohol?

A: Unfortunately some do, most don't.

Q: Most 12-year-olds don't go around growing marijuana?

A: Some do, most don't.

Q: Most of them don't harvest marijuana and sell it?

A: Some do, most don't.

Q: The answer is most don't. So what's the answer?

A: Yes.

Q: Most 12-year-olds don't maintain and use weapons and keep a weapon next to their bed?

A: Most don't.

Q: [After the alleged abuse by the police,] did he call the District Attorney's Office?

A: I doubt that Rudy Manzella would call the District Attorney's Office.

Q: Do you know?

A: He didn't. I know he didn't.

Q: Did he call Judge Kinsley in the City of Tonawanda?

A: No.

Q: Did he call Joel Daniels [defense counsel who was hired after the shootings]?

A: Why would he call Joel Daniels?

Q: Did he call him?

A: No.

Q: Did he call the Sheriff's Department?

A: No.

Q: Did he call Uncle Tony?

A: No.[34]

To rebut my testimony, the prosecution countered with that of Newman and Barton. I was surprised to see Newman called as a witness but not surprised that he essentially repudiated the results of the MMPI-2 he had given Rudy and earlier reported to the prosecutor without reservation or qualification. He explained that since some of the scaled MMPI-2 scores on the test he gave Rudy differed somewhat from those on the test I gave him, some of his findings now had to be interpreted with caution.

Predictably, Barton disagreed with my opinions in this case. With no training or experience in intelligence testing, and having administered no tests at all in this case, he opined that Rudy's IQ was in the normal range. The IQ of 82 that Rudy achieved in the testing I had done with him, Barton explained, was "attributable to the unethical conduct of Dr. Ewing in marking [Rudy's] answers too harshly."[35]

As expected, Barton also concluded that Rudy had not been in a state of extreme emotional disturbance when he shot the police officers. Instead, Barton told the jury that Rudy was "just a maladjusted, malevolent cop-hater who resented any restrictions of his activities."[36] Barton also testified that did not believe Rudy's accounts of the abuse by the officers in Tonawanda because at times Rudy answered inconsistently regarding how many officers were present at any given moment and because he was unable to precisely identify the room in which he had been abused.

On cross-examination, Barton admitted that he testified repeatedly for the district attorneys in at least seven local counties. In the five years preceding Rudy's trial, he acknowledged, in two of these counties alone he had been paid over $220,000 by prosecutors for his services.

Otherwise the cross-examination was much like that to which Barton had been exposed by defense attorney Joel Daniels several years earlier in the first trial of John Justice.

Despite my opinion that Rudy acted in extreme emotional disturbance when he shot the police officers and thus should have been convicted of manslaughter rather than murder, he was, as Barton had been quick to note, a cop-killer. Thus, I felt certain that the jury would not wrestle with the case very long and would convict him of murder and attempted murder as charged. Much to my surprise, however, after the jurors were instructed and began deliberating, it quickly became clear that they were, in fact, struggling with the issue of extreme emotional disturbance.

While deliberating, the jurors sent the judge a note that read: "The jury requests more instructions from the Judge. If a jury believes that the Defendant suffers from an emotional disturbance that influenced him to commit a crime, but the jury also believes that there are many other personality characteristics that are involved which may give him a tendency to commit criminal acts, may the jury still agree with a defense of extreme emotional disturbance? In other words, must the emotional disturbance be the only or overwhelming cause of the crime or may it be just one of several factors that led to the crime?"[37]

The judge responded as follows:

> The answer to your first question is that while you may believe or find that there are several factors that led this defendant to commit the crime as charged in the first four counts of the indictment; that is the murder counts, you are to consider whether the Defendant committed murder or attempted murder while influenced by an extreme emotional disturbance and whether that emotional disturbance was extreme and so influenced his conduct, that it caused him to lose such normal and rational self control as would otherwise influence his conduct.
>
> The emotional disturbance cannot be merely or just one of several factors which influenced his conduct leading to the crime. The emotional disturbance must be the overwhelming factor influencing his conduct at the time of the killing and attempted killing, to such an extent that his usual ability to control his conduct is impaired.[38]

The judge then reinstructed the jury regarding extreme emotional disturbance:

> First, you must determine whether this particular Defendant did in fact act under extreme emotional disturbance; that is at the time of the shootings was this Defendant's conduct influenced by his extreme emotional disturbance.
>
> After determining what the credible facts and circumstances are, and putting yourself in the defendant's shoes, under the facts and circumstances as he subjectively believed them to be, did he, in fact, act under the influence of extreme emotional disturbance, or, and that's part of your question, or did he act under some other, some other influence or for some other malevolent reason. Now, if he did, if he reacted under some other influence or for some other malevolent reason, then he did not act under the influence of extreme emotional disturbance. Your job is not to conclude with certainty what that other influence or reason might have been. But rather to decide whether, in fact, was defendant's conduct influenced by extreme emotional disturbance.[39]

Defense attorney Joel Daniels objected to this instruction, as it clearly misstated the law. New York's statute requires only that the defendant's conduct be influenced by an extreme emotional disturbance for which there is a reasonable excuse or explanation, not that the extreme emotional disturbance be the sole cause or even an "overwhelming" cause of the defendant's conduct.

Daniels's objection was overruled and the jury resumed deliberations. Ultimately the jurors convicted Rudy of murder and he was sentenced to 51 years to life in prison, 25 years for murder, 25 years for attempted murder and one year for obstructing governmental administration.

On appeal, even the prosecutor conceded that the one-year sentence for obstructing governmental administration could not be made consecutive to the other terms of incarceration. Thus, Rudy's sentence was reduced to 50 years to life. The appellate court, however, affirmed the convictions, holding that Rudy failed to prove that he acted under extreme emotional disturbance or that, if he did, there was a reasonable excuse or explanation for such a disturbance. Specifically, the court ruled that neither Rudy nor anyone else present at the time of the alleged police abuse testified as to what happened. The only evidence of that confrontation came from my testimony, the court said, and that was hearsay evidence admissible to provide the basis for my opinion regarding Rudy's state of mind but not to prove that the abuse actually occurred.

Subsequently the City of Tonawanda and its police department were sued by the son of the deputy who was killed and by the deputy who survived the shooting. The City settled with the dead deputy's son for an undisclosed amount of money. At trial, a jury awarded the surviving deputy \$2.4 million. At the same time, the civil jury awarded no damages against the detective Rudy claimed had been his primary abuser. Ultimately, the City, which was uninsured, paid the surviving deputy a sum of \$1.8 million in taxpayer dollars in full satisfaction of the \$2.4 million verdict and accrued interest.

CHAPTER 10

Insanity, Posttraumatic Stress Disorder, and Brief Reactive Psychosis

10

It sounded like an ordinary street robbery gone bad, so I was surprised to hear about it on National Public Radio's early morning hourly national newscast. The report out of Milwaukee was that a 17-year-old girl had shot and killed a 15-year-old girl over a leather coat. Sadly, at that time, such stories were so common in America's major cities that they were often unreported by the local media, and almost unheard of in national news reports.

But as I listened to NPR's report in more detail, I heard the teenager's court-appointed attorney give potentially greater meaning to the story. Robin Shellow, a top-notch criminal lawyer known for her spirited defense of children charged with crimes, explained that her young client, Felicia Morgan was innocent by reason of insanity. Okay, I thought instantly, that's still not national news. But then Shellow dropped the bomb: the diagnosis that would support Felicia's insanity defense was "urban psychosis."

As Shellow explained, Felicia, a victim of crime and child abuse, had grown up in a neighborhood where guns, assaults, robberies, and other violence were so common that she had lost her capacity to know what she was doing and that it was wrong.

I laughed out loud. It appeared to me that this was another one of those rare but striking cases in which a lawyer was attempting to plead what I had for years been telling my students was the "rotten life defense."

I stopped laughing a few days later when I got a call from Shellow, asking me to come to Milwaukee, examine Felicia, and see if I agreed that she was insane at the time of the robbery-murder. She had chosen to call me, she said, because I had recently written two books dealing with juvenile homicide, *When Children Kill* and *Kids Who Kill.*[1] I had also worked on a number of other juvenile homicide cases in Wisconsin.

I quickly dismissed any notion of "urban psychosis," but was intrigued by Shellow's thumbnail analysis of her client and realized that even if there was no such thing as "urban psychosis," that did not mean that Felicia Morgan might not be legally insane.

Robin Shellow is one of the most persuasive and tenacious lawyers with whom I have ever worked. While she could not sell me on urban psychosis—I suspect that she did not even intend to—she had certainly gotten my attention and convinced me to at least consider examining her young client. I would review the file and decide whether it was worth examining Felicia. Even if I decided to do so, I did not expect much to come of my evaluation. I had rarely found a defendant to be legally insane and, even then, juries were rarely persuaded. At that point in my career, I had completed insanity evaluations of approximately 46 homicide defendants and had found just 3 to be legally insane at the time of their offenses.

By the time I got involved in the case, Felicia had been through a lengthy court proceeding in which a judge decided that she should be tried as an adult rather than as a juvenile. As part of that proceeding, Felicia had been evaluated by four other local psychologists. Their reports were included in the file I reviewed, as were the results of their psychological testing. Those reports, coupled with all the other evidence available in the case, convinced me that Felicia was a seriously troubled youngster who had gone through a horrific childhood and whose behavior at the time of the shooting might well have been influenced by her tragic history and obvious mental health problems. At the very least, these records certainly indicated that what Robin Shellow told me was no exaggeration.

Even though the records were detailed and graphic and I expected Felicia to be extremely disturbed, I was still surprised by what I found when I went to the jail in Milwaukee and examined her. Much of the six-hour nonstop interview resembled a living nightmare in which I not only heard about—but actually saw evidence of—the horror that had been done to this child and the pain, fear, and desperation that it had caused.

Having evaluated thousands of troubled and distressed individuals in the course of my career, I have seen pretty much the full gamut of human emotion: everything from the deepest anguish and remorse to icy, psychopathic indifference. I have spent hours with defendants who could barely speak through their pain and tears and similar amounts of time with unrepentant, stone-faced killers, who described their crimes as though recounting a favorite movie or television program.

At times, Felicia's speech was logical, rational, and coherent but she was constantly moving and hypervigilant, always looking over her shoulder, easily distracted, tense, and paranoid. At times, she lapsed into what appeared to be an uncontrollable rocking behavior. When discussing some of the abuse she had suffered as a child and adolescent, she entered a trancelike state in which she carried on conversations with others who were not present. When I pressed her about the abuse, she became agitated, rambling, and almost incoherent. When I tried to press her to be more responsive and pushed for more information at a number of points in the examination, Felicia rolled onto the floor, screamed, cried, and banged her body against the wall. In what is now a 30-plus-year career as a forensic psychologist, I have never seen a patient this distraught, hysterical, and dissociated.

It took all day, but I was finally able to obtain a detailed history from Felicia and her account of what happened on the night of the killing.

Felicia had grown up in an environment of extreme family and neighborhood violence. At home, from childhood through her early teenage years, she had often been beaten by her mother with extension cords, leather belts, switches, and other objects. Her mother had threatened to kill her and had once put a knife to her throat, telling Felicia, "I put you in this world and I can take you out."[2] Throughout her childhood and adolescence, her mother also abused her psychologically, calling her a "bitch," "whore," "slut," "tramp," "bastard," "motherfucker," and a host of other degrading names.[3]

Felicia had also been abused by her grandparents and her older sister. Her grandfather whipped her with a belt, often to the point that she was too bruised to attend school. Her grandmother also whipped her but, according to Felicia, "only if it was necessary."[4] When Felicia was four or five years old, her sister burned Felicia's arm with a hot iron, leaving a scar that was still visible when I saw her over a decade later.

Felicia also witnessed a great deal of domestic violence between her parents. When Felicia was three, her father fired a gun at her mother "because there was too much salt in the gravy."[5] From age four to about age six, Felicia often watched her parents eat dinner with loaded guns at their sides, each feeling the need to protect himself or herself from the other.

Felicia had also been sexually abused as a child and adolescent. As a child, she was molested by a man who was giving her a bath. When her mother realized what was happening, she shot the man in front of Felicia. As a 14-year-old, Felicia was raped by the son of her family's landlord.

Felicia was also no stranger to gun violence, criminal victimization, and homicide. In addition to watching her parents use firearms in the home, Felicia and a number of her relatives and friends had been shot or threatened with shooting. In 1987, Felicia was robbed and severely beaten by a gang of girls. In 1988, Felicia stepped in front of a man with a gun in an effort to protect her aunt. Later that year, Felicia's cousin was shot in a street fight and left with a paralyzed arm. In 1989, Felicia was again robbed at gunpoint.

In September 1990, Felicia's uncle (a close friend) was shot and killed. A month later, her cousin was killed in a drive-by shooting. In

December 1990, Felicia was robbed of her coat at gunpoint. The next month, January 1991, the boyfriend of Felicia's sister, a man who was a surrogate father to Felicia, was shot and paralyzed. In September 1991, just a month before she killed 15-year-old Brenda Adams, Felicia was again robbed by a gang of girls.

Three weeks before the killing, gang members shot at a friend in Felicia's presence. No more than a week later, and just about two weeks before the killing, a man pulled a gun on Felicia, her mother, and a friend. Felicia stepped in front of the gunman, protecting her mother and friend until her mother intervened to defuse the threat.

The killing of Brenda Adams was the culmination of a 15-minute crime spree that occurred early on the morning of October 26, 1991. Felicia and 15-year-old Manuella "Marie" Johnson were riding to a party in a car driven by Kurearte "K-Dog" Oliver, an older male friend. The trio passed three men on the street, one of whom hollered to K-Dog, "You see that white bitch back there? She got on a herringbone, dog."[6] In street parlance, the man was telling K-Dog that the young woman was wearing a gold herringbone necklace. K-Dog responded by handing Felicia a small-caliber handgun and telling her and Marie to "get the herringbone for me."[7]

Felicia and Marie got out of the car and started toward the girl with the necklace. Suddenly, the three men reappeared, shoved Felicia and Marie aside, grabbed the girl's necklace, and ran away. Felicia and Marie retreated to the car and Felicia told K-Dog, "Them dudes beat me to it and got the herringbone."[8] Felicia, Marie, and K-Dog then drove away in search of the three men.

Soon, they saw three girls and a boy on the street. They stopped and asked if the youths had seen the three men. Their reply was negative and, as K-Dog started to drive away, Marie said she wanted the coat that one of the girls was wearing. She and Felicia exited the car and confronted the youths. Felicia pointed the gun at them. Then she and Marie took a necklace, a coat and a baseball cap from them.

Felicia and Marie rejoined K-Dog, who drove them to the party they had been planning to attend. From the car, Marie saw Brenda Adams standing outside the apartment in which the party was being held. She pointed to Brenda's leather coat and said, "I want that trench."[9] K-Dog pulled the car around the corner and Felicia and Marie got out. Before Felicia could shut the car door, K-Dog handed her the gun and said, "Let Marie do what she got to do and don't let no niggers get into it."[10]

Felicia and Marie crossed the street and directed Brenda to give them her coat. When Brenda refused, Marie started fighting with her. Others began to gather around the altercation and Felicia brandished the firearm and told them to keep their distance. Felicia and Marie fought with Brenda and eventually Marie dragged her across the street. As Brenda lay slumped against a light pole, Felicia pointed the gun in her direction and fired one shot into her shoulder. Felicia and Marie made off with Brenda's coat, ran back to K-Dog's car, and left the scene. Meanwhile Brenda died from the gunshot wound.

Later that day, Felicia turned herself in to the police. Felicia told officers that after Marie dragged Brenda across the street, she heard shots being fired from across the street, shut her eyes and fired a single shot. According to Felicia's account, when she opened her eyes, her arm was pointed at Brenda's shoulder. She said that she helped Marie take Brenda's coat and then grabbed Brenda's necklace, adding that when she saw blood on Brenda's shoulder she dropped the necklace. Felicia told the police that when she was approaching the car, she heard additional gunshots from across the street, to which she responded by turning back and firing another shot at Brenda.

Facing charges that included five armed robberies, one attempted armed robbery, and a murder, forced to stand trial as an adult, and confronting the possibility of spending the rest of her life in prison, Felicia had pleaded not guilty by reason of insanity. In Wisconsin, that meant that potentially she faced a two-phase trial. In the first phase, a jury would determine her guilt or innocence without regard to insanity. If she were convicted, she would then have the opportunity in a second phase to present her insanity defense.

Following my examination of Felicia, I was not ready to make a diagnosis of urban psychosis, but I could see clearly what Robin Shellow meant when she put that label on her young client months earlier. Felicia suffered from long-standing posttraumatic stress disorder (PTSD) as a result of the abuse and criminal victimization she had experienced and witnessed throughout her life. Among the symptoms of PTSD Felicia presented were hypervigilance (i.e., constantly fearing and literally being on the lookout for something horrible to happen to her); difficulty concentrating; flashbacks in which she psychologically reexperienced the earlier traumas; and frequent intrusive and unwanted thoughts of the prior traumas.

Based on my examination of Felicia and all the evidence I reviewed, I also concluded that, at the time of the homicide, she was suffering from a brief reactive psychosis.

The then-applicable *Diagnostic and Statistical Manual of Mental Disorders,* Third Edition—Revised (known as the *DSM-III-R*) described brief reactive psychosis as follows:

> The essential feature of this disorder is sudden onset of psychotic symptoms of at least a few hours', but no more than one month's, duration, with eventual full return to premorbid level of functioning. The psychotic symptoms appear shortly after one or more events that, singly or together, would be markedly stressful to almost anyone in similar circumstances in that person's culture. The precipitating event(s) may be any major stress, such as the loss of a loved one or the psychological trauma of combat. Invariably there is emotional turmoil, manifested by rapid shifts from one intense affect to another, or overwhelming perplexity or confusion, which the person may acknowledge or which can be judged from the way he or she responds to questions and requests.[11]

The *DSM-III-R* added that "[t]he disorder usually appears in adolescence or early adulthood" and listed specific symptoms that must have been present in order to make the diagnosis.[12]

In Felicia's case, the requisite psychotic symptoms she showed at and around the time of the homicide included impaired reality testing, delusions, hallucinations, and disorganized behavior.

In my view, Felicia's past experience—both personal and vicarious—with abuse and criminal victimization left her vulnerable to the stresses she encountered on the street the night of the killing: being directed to take part in robberies, taking part in robberies, finding herself with a gun in her hand in what was almost a war zone, and hearing gunshots fired nearby. My ultimate forensic conclusion was that, as a result of PTSD and the brief reactive psychosis she experienced that night, Felicia was, at the time she shot Brenda Adams, substantially unable to appreciate the wrongfulness of her actions and to conform her conduct to the requirements of law. In short, my opinion was that Felicia was insane at the time of the killing.

Since I had reached such a conclusion, Shellow asked me to testify at trial on Felicia's behalf. Only after she had secured my opinion, did Shellow divulge to me that she had also had Felicia examined by another psychologist with expertise in juvenile homicide, Dr. Dewey Cornell, a clinical psychologist, professor at the University of Virginia, and coeditor of the book, *Juvenile Homicide*.[13] Unknown to me, and completely independent of my examination, Dr. Cornell had reviewed the evidence, examined Felicia, and diagnosed her as suffering from PTSD and a borderline personality disorder. According to the *DSM-III-R:*

> The essential feature of [borderline personality] disorder is a pervasive pattern of instability of self-image, interpersonal relationships, and mood. . . .
>
> A marked and persistent identity disturbance is almost invariably present. . . .
>
> Interpersonal relationships are usually unstable and intense. . . .
>
> Affective instability is common. This may be evidenced by marked mood shifts from baseline mood to depression, irritability or anxiety, usually lasting a few hours or, only rarely, more than a few days. In addition these people often have inappropriately intense anger, with frequent displays of temper or recurrent physical fights. They tend to be impulsive, particularly in activities that are potentially self-damaging. . . .
>
> [They may experience] feelings of "numbness" and depersonalization that arise during periods of extreme stress. . . .

> During periods of extreme stress, transient psychotic symptoms may occur, but they are generally of insufficient severity or duration to warrant an additional diagnosis.[14]

Also, unknown to me prior to my evaluation, Shellow had asked Dr. James Garbarino to consult on the case. Garbarino, who was not a clinician but an internationally renowned developmental psychologist and expert on the causes of juvenile violence, did not examine Felicia but reviewed the evidence in the case, including Felicia's history.

Shellow believed that my testimony and that of Garbarino belonged in both phases of the trial, the innocence-guilt proceeding and the insanity proceeding. She believed that our testimony would undermine one of the essential elements of the case the prosecution had to prove to convict Felicia of murder: intent to kill. As she argued to the trial judge:

> Dr. Ewing has examined the defendant and will offer testimony about the defendant's mental health condition. He will testify that as a result of his examination of Felicia Morgan and six hours of interviews, his diagnosis is that Felicia Morgan suffers from Posttraumatic Stress Disorder and Brief Reactive Psychosis. Dr. Ewing will also testify to the effects of PTSD on its victims and resulting symptoms, including "flashback" dissociative states and hypervigilance. . . .
>
> A second expert, Dr. James Garbarino, will also offer testimony necessary to assist the jury in understanding PTSD and the effects that mental disorder has on its sufferers. . . . As the leading national research scientist on the effects of violence on children, Dr. Garbarino will testify as to the current state of research and its applicability to children like Felicia Morgan who live in violent communities and are witnesses and victims to excessive violence.[15]

Unimpressed with these arguments, the judge refused to allow us to testify at the guilt-innocence phase of the trial and told Shellow in court:

> I think the bottom line is Wisconsin does not allow testimony detailing psychiatric and personal history in the first phase except under very limited circumstances which I have talked about. . . . So the court would

> rule that this type of material or testimony will not be allowed during the first phase of this trial. . . . No irrelevant social testimony. Definitely no experts are going to come in. I don't know what I can say about lay [witnesses]. You have family members that are going to talk about something that may be relevant to the issue of intent, I can't anticipate what that would be. But if it's with this fact that she is, has this trauma, even her life where she's been exposed to all this violence, so therefore, she—whether she was confronted with the situation, she did something she didn't intend to do, then it's irrelevant on that issue, yes. No lay or expert testimony on that issue.[16]

As Shellow saw it, although the court's ruling did not preclude Felicia from testifying, it did exclude any testimony regarding PTSD and flashbacks the young defendant might have had at the time of the killing. As Shellow put it, Felicia "could testify that she did not intend to kill Brenda Adams" but the court's ruling "silenced her explanation as to why she did not intend to kill Brenda Adams."[17]

Faced with this adverse ruling from the trial judge, Shellow chose to present no evidence in the first phase of the trial. After hearing only the prosecution's case, the jury found Felicia guilty on all counts charged, including first degree murder. Only then did Felicia have the chance to present a meaningful defense.

During the second phase of her trial, Felicia testified as to her own mental state at the time of the killing:

Q: Lisa, when you heard—did you hear voices on October 26, 1991?

A: Yes.

Q: Were these when you were sleeping or when you were awake?

A: I was awake.

Q: When is the first time you heard voices on October 26, 1991?

A: When we—when we saw three girls and the boy.

Q: And where did the voices come from?

A: I can't really describe it. It was—

Q: Try. The jury needs to know. Try.

A: It is kind of hard. It is hard for me to describe. It was—

Q: Well.

A: It was when I recognized the one girl that helped jump on me, you know, he—that voice. You know, I just picked it off from her and the girls that jumped on me and, you know, the voice was like, Yeah, she took your stuff. You take hers.

Q: And when is the next time that you heard a voice on October 26, 1991?

A: Um, when I was—I had let them two dudes—I had them two dudes off me, and they like went cross the street. And I was walking backwards across the street. And something, you know—that voice just said, Look up. And I looked up.

Q: And what did you see when you looked up?

A: It was a dude standing in the window.

Q: And was this in a first-story or second-story window?

A: Second story. It was, you know, in the upstairs.

Q: What did he look like?

A: I don't know. All I know he was black, and he had a black gun.

Q: And what's the next thing that—the next voice that you heard after the black man with the black gun in the window?

A: I put my hand back down.

The Court: You have to speak up, please.

A: I pulled my hand back down because I—at the time I had reached the corner, but that voice just said, Look back up again. Look back up, and I looked up and—I looked up.

Q: Was he still there?

A: Who?

Q: The man in the window.

A: No, he was outside.

Q: And do you remember being shot at on October 26, 1991?

A: Yes.

Q: When were you shot at?

A: When that voice told me the second time to look back up, that's when he shot me again.

Q: And did you tell Dr. Ewing or Dr. Cornell that you thought you were hit?

A: Yes.

Q: Why did you think you were hit?

A: I started—my eyes started to rolling in my head, and I was spinning like sideways, frontwards and backwards. I was feeling—I was real weakish, and my eyes and stuff was rolling.

Q: Were you shot on October 26, 1991?

A: No.

Q: You went and—after Brenda Adams was shot, Lisa, do you know if you killed Brenda Adams?

A: No, I don't know.

Q: There has been—you've heard all of the testimony in this case; right?

A: Yes.

Q: Do you think you killed Brenda Adams?

A: I don't know.

Q: You heard Marie talk about leaning over and shooting Brenda Adams at point-blank range?

A: Yes, I heard it.

Q: Did that convince you that you killed Brenda Adams?

A: I don't know.[18]

As promised in Shellow's pretrial motion, I testified that Felicia suffered from PTSD and was suffering a brief reactive psychosis at the time of the killing. Specifically I testified that she had been experiencing delusions, hallucinations, and disorganized behavior.

With regard to delusions, I testified:

> A delusion is a belief that something has happened, is happening or is going on or is about to happen that flies in the face of what other people know to be the truth. An example of a delusion in this case—I thought I was shot....
>
> Ms. Morgan indicated to me that at the time immediately preceding the shooting of Ms. Adams that she believed she had been shot. She clearly wasn't shot, but to believe that in the face of all the evidence that she doesn't have a bullet in her, that she is not bleeding, that she is not injured, is delusional....
>
> That I think is the—the only delusion at that particular moment, at the time of the shooting, but preceding the shooting there was another incident in which she robbed another girl and she—Ms. Morgan was convinced that this girl absolutely beyond a doubt had previously robbed her and assaulted her. This delusion was so rigid and so fixed and so extremely held by her that when I confronted her with the fact that this couldn't possibly have been the girl, she argued with me, she screamed, she yelled. She became almost incoherent trying to defend her position that, yes, this was the same girl who had in fact robbed her earlier. That's a delusion. It is a fixed belief in something that can't possibly be true and has been demonstrated, I understand it, right here in court, to be [false].[19]

With regard to hallucinations, I told the jury:

> A hallucination is a perception of something as real when it is not real. Hallucinations can be visual, seeing things that aren't there, auditory, hearing voices or hearing things that aren't there. There are tactile hallucinations, feeling things that aren't there. There are even olfactory hallucinations, smelling things, and gustatory hallucinations, tasting things that are not there....
>
> The most common kind, that is auditory hallucinations. At the time of the confrontation with the robbery victim whom she believed to have robbed her, she heard a voice telling her—I have to look at my report to get the precise words.... [S]he approached this girl and the voice said

> words to the effect of pay back, pay back. She stole your shit. Now steal her shit. She heard a voice in her head. . . .
>
> At the time of the actual shooting she heard a voice telling her to look up, and she didn't tell me this but she told another examiner, I believe, that she heard voices saying other things around the time of the actual killing.[20]

With regard to disorganized behavior at or near the time of the killing, I testified: "Well it can be anything from wildly flailing about in a disorganized fashion to just very unconventional, deviant or bizarre behavior. What Ms. Morgan recounted to me was that as she began to hear gunshots at around the time just before the shooting of Ms. Adams, that she developed what I guess would best be described as kind of a wobbling posture that she couldn't control. It is kind of hard for me to describe it verbally. Perhaps I could—"[21]

With the court's indulgence, I physically demonstrated the odd rocking behavior Felicia had described to me and had shown at times of extreme stress in my examination.

On cross-examination, the prosecutor followed the general script for trying to discredit expert psychological testimony. She asked if PTSD and brief reactive psychosis were diseases and got me to agree that, while I believed they were, there is controversy in the mental health field as to what constitutes an illness, disorder, or disease. Then, instead of challenging the diagnoses I had made, she tried to make light of the *DSM-III-R,* noting that in that encyclopedic volume nicotine dependence and alcohol dependence were classified as disorders.

The prosecutor also got me to acknowledge, as I routinely do, that if any of the facts I relied on in formulating my opinion were proven false, then I might change my opinion. Even then, however, I stressed that while some of the facts in this case were in question, what mattered more to me psychologically was what Felicia perceived at the time she shot and killed Brenda Adams.

More fruitfully, the prosecutor got me to acknowledge, as I had to, that given the somewhat confusing sequence of events on the night of the killing, it was impossible to say precisely when Felicia became psychotic. As I went on to testify: "My opinion goes to the homicide. I am not clear about that preceding robbery, the robbery in which the girl looked like or reminded or made her think she was the girl who had robbed her earlier. And I can't really render an opinion about that because [of] the very thing you've pointed out. The sequence is so unclear. Did she rob her and then become convinced that it was the girl, or did she start to rob her and become convinced, or did she become convinced and then rob her? It is not entirely clear."[22]

Dr. Cornell's testimony followed mine. He testified that in his expert opinion Felicia suffered from PTSD, borderline personality disorder, and brief reactive psychosis at the time of the offenses, and that as a result she could not appreciate the wrongfulness of her actions. He went on to explain that "individuals with a Borderline Personality Disorder are prone to have brief psychotic episodes" and gave the jury his definition of psychosis: "Psychosis is a broad term that isn't a specific disorder, but it refers to a level of functioning in which the person is not in complete contact with reality, in which the person might be having hallucinations; that is, false perception such as hearing voices. They might have delusions such as a paranoid belief that somebody is out to get them, which is an unshakeable belief."[23]

Shellow attempted to get Dr. Garbarino's testimony before the jury but was stymied when the judge ruled that it was irrelevant and a "waste of time."[24] In order to preserve the testimony for the record in the event of an appeal, Shellow was allowed to present Garbarino's proposed testimony outside the hearing of the jury. Garbarino described the development of PTSD in children placed in extremely violent or stressful situations. Unlike my testimony or that of Cornell, Garbarino focused on the exposure of children to violence in war zones and likened their plight and pathological responses to those of urban youths who, like Felicia, had repeatedly witnessed and experienced extreme violence at home and in the streets of their communities.

Ten of the twelve jurors rejected Felicia's insanity defense. Despite the lack of unanimity, under Wisconsin law she was thus criminally responsible for all of the charges the jurors had previously found proven beyond a reasonable doubt. Now all that was left was the sentence to be imposed. For many reasons, I expected Felicia to receive the harshest sentence the law would allow. Foremost among these reasons was the apparent attitude of the trial judge toward Felicia, her defense, and the psychologists, including me, who supported that defense in court.

The trial judge, Michael Guolee, had not only refused to allow expert testimony in the guilt-innocence phase of the trial and excluded Dr. Garbarino's testimony altogether, but later made a number of disparaging remarks that appeared directed at the experts in this case, myself included, the defense attorney, and the defendant. He said, apparently referring to the *DSM-III-R*, "Attorneys are confronted with a terrible situation and a terrible fact situation. They have no real defense, so when they look into this book and they find something, they say, 'Hey, this is good, I can use this.' And then they'll find a psychiatrist who'll say, 'Yeah, I can do that.' "[25] He added, "I don't know why people come to my court the way they come here, and I can't be involved in that and the law can't be involved in that. We cannot be social scientists. We have to set standards and those standards have to be followed."[26] With regard to Felicia, he stated, "She's just an antisocial person. I have hundreds like this that come into my courts. She's not any different than any of them."[27]

Near the end of my cross-examination, Guolee threatened to have me jailed if I did not return to court the next day to complete my testimony. As I was testifying that day in Milwaukee, both attorneys and the judge knew that I was under subpoena to testify in another murder trial the next morning in Buffalo. Shortly after 5:00 PM, with less than two hours to go before the departure of the last flight that would get me to Buffalo by the next morning, my cross-examination was virtually complete. Suddenly, the judge ordered a short recess.

During the break, I reminded him of my predicament, produced the New York subpoena, and asked if we could forgo the recess and instead complete my testimony so I might make my flight. Guolee told me that the subpoena was my problem. When I got up and put on my overcoat to leave for the airport, he directed me to sit down or face jail for contempt of court. I sat down, removed my coat, waited through the recess, and then listened as the judge told the jury that my testimony would be completed neither then nor the next day but the day after that, which was a Saturday. Unhappy to be forced to fly back to Milwaukee the next night but relieved that I could meet my obligation in Buffalo, I hurried from the courtroom, rushed to the airport, and caught my flight. When I arrived in Buffalo later that evening, a message from the judge awaited me: I would be allowed to finish my testimony the following Monday via telephone. I did so in a matter of minutes.

The prosecution had asked the judge to sentence Felicia to a term of 60 years to life in prison. Even at her young age, that could be a life sentence. I anticipated that the judge would accede to the prosecutor's request and was surprised when instead of imposing the harshest sentence, he imposed the most lenient sentence possible under the law. Guolee sentenced Felicia to a life sentence with no minimum, which automatically made her eligible for parole in 13 years and four months.

Felicia's conviction was appealed to a state appellate court, which affirmed the conviction. The appeals court found no error in refusing expert testimony during the guilt-innocence phase of the trial, concluding that the "mere diagnosis" of PTSD did not support any recognized defense or serve to refute any specific element of the offenses with which Felicia was charged.[28] However, as one member of the court noted in dissent:

> The majority contradicts its own acknowledgment of Morgan's theory of defense when it claims that she offered only "the mere diagnosis of posttraumatic stress disorder as a 'blanket' defense" but did not do so either to refute a specific element of the offense or to support a recognized defense. That assertion is inconsistent with the record. In the first place, as noted, Morgan offered not "the mere diagnosis" of PTSD, but rather, the diagnosis in combination with its actual *causation* of her actions. In the second place, just as the majority had conceded earlier, Morgan attempted to offer PTSD evidence both to refute a specific element—intent, and to support a recognized defense—lack of intent.[29]

The majority of the state appeals court held that the trial court erred in finding Dr. Garbarino's testimony irrelevant but concluded that it was properly excluded as cumulative because it duplicated aspects of my testimony and that of Dr. Cornell. Even the dissenting judge felt constrained to agree that the trial judge had the discretion to exclude Garbarino's testimony. Still, he added, "I would hope, nevertheless, that judges and policymakers everywhere will become familiar with Dr. Garbarino's extraordinary research and writing. Dr. Garbarino's work is more than 'relevant.' His scholarship exposes the devastation of children throughout the world, pierces the conscience of those who are able to shed denial, and motivates all who will listen, learn, and fight for the protection of children."[30]

Finally, the appellate court then went out of its way to gratuitously condemn Felicia's defense, even going so far as to cite evidence (a magazine article) not contained anywhere in the record:

> While she does not use the phrase in her appellate brief, Morgan's counsel has elsewhere used the phrase "urban psychosis" to describe her criminal defense theory for Morgan's actions in Adams's homicide. . . . We reach no conclusions on the psychiatric accuracy or clinical reliability of such a term, but note that we are unable to locate any academic or judicial support for, or recognition of, such an "urban psychosis" defense. Accordingly, this court will not be the first to give such recognition to an unfounded legal concept.[31]

Again the dissenting judge took issue with the majority's view, pointing out that, as a matter of fact, "[a]lthough the media may have offered insightful and provocative commentary using these words, the record establishes that Morgan did not pursue any theory of defense in these specific terms."[32]

Many if not most criminal convictions would have ended with the final decision of the state's appellate court, but Robin Shellow turned next to the federal courts, claiming that the trial court's refusal to allow me and Dr. Garbarino to testify during the guilt-innocence phase of the trial, violated Felicia's federal constitutional right to defend herself. A federal district court judge in Milwaukee read and heard arguments in the case, agreed with Shellow, and ordered a new trial for Felicia. Judge Lynn Adelman concluded, among other things:

> The goal of Morgan's proffer was to introduce evidence casting doubt on the state's essential contention that when she pulled the trigger she had "a purpose" to kill Brenda Adams or was aware that her conduct was "practically certain to cause that result." Under Wisconsin's statutory homicide scheme, negating this intent element diminishes the state's charge from first-degree intentional homicide to first-degree reckless homicide. . . .
>
> Morgan's motions *in limine* provided a somewhat more vivid description of her alleged dissociative state than the court of appeals appears to credit. Morgan did not merely claim that the *fact* of her dissociation rendered her incapable of intending to kill. She claimed that when she heard the gunshots she was scared, that she was swaying back and forth and felt as if she were going to pass out . . . that her eyes got heavy and she felt as if she were in a trance . . . that her reaction to the gunfire of others occurred only moments before she is alleged to have shot Brenda Adams . . . that she does not remember shooting Brenda Adams. . . . The overwhelming claim that emerges from the proffers' numerous references to Morgan's mental condition at the moment of the killing is that she was in a "trance-like" state when the gun went off. In common understanding, this description connotes a dazed, somnolent, almost hypnotic state. It is difficult to understand how a defendant's trance-like dissociation from her immediate surroundings, if true, would *not* be relevant to the likelihood that she formed an intent to kill or was aware that her conduct was certain to have that result. . . .
>
> In sum, the court of appeals concluded that Morgan's theory of defense was not relevant to her intent to kill either because of an erroneous or incomplete understanding of her alleged dissociative state at the time of the homicide, or because of an erroneous belief that [Wisconsin case law] renders inadmissible all or nearly all psychiatric evidence offered to disprove a defendant's capacity to intend. Based on clear Wisconsin precedent and a "common-sense understanding" that a defendant's trance-like condition at the time of a killing may be highly probative of her intent to kill, Morgan's PTSD theory of defense was relevant in the guilt phase of her trial. . . .

> [A]lthough the trial court expressed its general distrust of Morgan's PTSD defense theory, her proffer was not excludable on that basis. The court made no finding that Morgan's experts were not qualified "by knowledge, skill, experience, training, or education." Indeed, two psychologists who examined Morgan and diagnosed her as suffering from PTSD were permitted to testify in the "responsibility" phase of her bifurcated trial, and another expert whose testimony was excluded as cumulative had impressive credentials. For that matter, even if Wisconsin trial judges were obligated or permitted to conduct a direct evaluation of the reliability of the proposed scientific theory, none was conducted here. Morgan's expert testimony was offered through qualified witnesses who used accepted diagnostic classification systems.[33]

Though the federal court decision was a clear victory for Felicia, it was short-lived. The prosecution appealed that decision to the U.S. Court of Appeals for the Seventh Circuit, which reversed it. The Seventh Circuit concluded:

> It is obvious that Judge Guolee, the state trial judge, wrestled with Morgan's proffer, cited appropriate case law, and ultimately determined that, given Wisconsin's skepticism about psychiatric testimony, much of Morgan's evidence should be excluded. He showed concern for Morgan's right to present a defense, but he also correctly noted that normally a defendant must rely on a recognizable defense—that there are "certain parameters as to defenses." He referred to the struggle the Wisconsin appellate courts have had in evaluating psychiatric testimony and their conclusion that such testimony often goes to a moral issue, which is the relevant inquiry in the second stage of a bifurcated trial. As to whether an expert might be allowed to testify to matters stopping short of the ultimate issue of capacity to form intent, the judge recognized the very "real dilemma" for a court in drawing and enforcing the boundaries between the two types of evidence. He then made clear that Morgan's own testimony was relevant as to what she was doing at the moment of the killing and why she "closed her eyes," for instance. When pressed as to whether he was excluding entirely the other lay testimony about the 17 incidents of trauma, he said, "That's pretty broad." He said he was excluding "irrelevant social testimony" but that he could not "anticipate

> what that would be," thus leaving the door open to some testimony, the precise contours of which would be determined as the evidence was presented. It was this ruling that the Wisconsin Court of Appeals affirmed. Even if it were our role to agree or disagree with this conclusion, we cannot say the court made the wrong call. And that's what it means to give "discretion" to the trial judge on evidentiary calls.
>
> As an aside, we note that Morgan would have placed a very heavy burden on the trial were she allowed to present 17 separate incidents of past traumatic incidents, some dating back to when she was a little girl. For instance (according to her pretrial submissions), she wanted to offer, through testimony of friends and family, that when she was "four to six years old, [she] witnessed her mother and father regularly dine with loaded revolvers at their sides during family dinners so that neither one would be unprotected from the violent outbursts of the other." She also wanted to show that her "cousin was shot in a 1988 street fight and subsequently lost the use of her arm" and that her mother "shot a man, in front of Morgan, because he was molesting Morgan while giving her a bath." We mentioned earlier that she also wanted to offer evidence that when she was only 3 years old, her father shot her mother "because there was too much salt in the gravy."
>
> Unless Morgan assumed the State would just sit back and listen to all this testimony without investigating its accuracy, she was in effect asking the trial judge to hold 17 mini-trials on collateral events, some of which were far outside any conceivably relevant time period.[34]

Though I am hardly an unbiased observer in this matter, I believe that the trial judge, the state court of appeals, and the Seventh Circuit were wrong and that the federal judge who remanded the case for a new trial was right. I am less certain about Dr. Garbarino's testimony, but I know that my testimony in this case would have gone directly to the issue of whether Felicia intended to kill Brenda Adams when she shot her. The prosecution knew of the proffered testimony well in advance and, if they had chosen, they certainly had the resources to investigate the truth of the claims made by Felicia and others regarding her victimization and exposure to violence. As far as I know, they never even bothered to look into these claims and certainly made no effort to disprove any of them, all of which were clearly pertinent to the diagnoses both Dr. Cornell and I tendered.

Despite the great controversy generated by this case and the slings and arrows Dr. Cornell, Dr. Garbarino, and I suffered as a result of our participation, I have never regretted my decision to enter the case. Nor have I ever doubted the diagnoses or the insanity determination that I reached. I was not a lawyer or an advocate in this case and had nothing riding on its outcome. Like Drs. Cornell and Garbarino, I carefully and conscientiously weighed all the evidence, applied the best teachings of my profession, called it as I saw it, honestly presented my conclusions, and willingly acknowledged their limitations when cross-examined. In my view, nothing more—and, of course, nothing less—could have been demanded of us.

Lessons Learned

What lessons can be gleaned from the 10 cases in this book? Although these cases are not presented as a representative sample of the work of forensic psychologists, or even representative examples of my own work, they illustrate points that I and others have often made about expert testimony in the field of forensic psychology.

First, these cases amply illustrate a seeming truism, but one that is sometimes ignored by experts, attorneys, judges, and jurors: expert opinions are opinions, not facts. As was seen in all these cases, my own opinions and those of my colleagues, though accepted by the courts as expert in nature, were challenged by other experts who had different, often polar opposite, opinions. It would be misleading and unfair to the field of forensic psychology if the reader were to take from this book the message that this is the only field or even one of a few fields in which this routinely happens. The fact is that in virtually every forensic field from forensic accounting to forensic zoology, experts often disagree when confronted with the same set of facts in the same case.

Part of the reason for these frequent "battles of the experts" is that these professionals are giving opinions—they are looking at a set of facts, applying their education, knowledge, and experience to those facts, and stating what are always, to one degree or another, subjective judgments. Courts are aware of this and have special rules to deal with expert testimony, including instructions to jurors that they are not bound by an expert's conclusion and are to judge the credibility of an expert like that of any other witness. Consider, for example, the court's lengthy jury instruction on weighing expert testimony in the Jimmy Lee Rouse case (Chapter 3).

A related explanation for the "battle of the experts" in forensic psychology and all other forensic disciplines is that experts are not required to be absolutely sure of their opinions. Courts have long recognized that a rule requiring absolute certainty would preclude almost all expert testimony, even that regarding such relatively clear-cut issues as DNA or fingerprint evidence. All that courts require from experts is that they be reasonably certain of their opinions before being allowed to offer them in court. Rarely does the law define the term reasonable or reasonably in any context. So, as a practical matter, experts are left to their professional and personal consciences in determining whether their opinions meet the standard of reasonable certainty.

Still another possible reason for the divergence of opinion in some cases is more sinister. Occasionally—not often, but at the same time too often—experts are essentially "hired guns." They are known to sell their testimony and command very high prices for the opinions they present in court. They are often repeat performers who become virtual employees of the attorneys or agencies for whose clients they present evidence.

In my experience, the hired gun phenomenon is exacerbated by certain legal rules, especially in criminal cases. In these cases, the conclusions of experts who evaluate a defendant for the defense are generally not required to be divulged to the prosecution unless the defense attorney plans to call the expert as a witness. Thus, if I examine a defendant for a defense attorney and, as usually happens, my conclusion does not support the defense position in the case, the defense attorney is free to discard my opinion and turn to one or more other experts looking for a favorable opinion. Not so for prosecutors. If an expert examines a criminal defendant at the behest of a prosecutor and reaches a conclusion that is favorable to the defense, the prosecutor has a legal duty to inform defense counsel of the expert's conclusion. In many cases where that occurs, the prosecution is then virtually forced to concede the psychological defense raised by the defendant. Thus, often, as a practical matter, prosecutors are much more likely than defense attorneys to seek conclusions from experts with a known track record if not a clear bias in favor of the prosecution.

A second lesson to be learned from the cases presented here is not as obvious as the first. Expert witnesses are frequently used in controversial, difficult, and high-profile cases, many of which could go either way. They are highly sought-after, generally well-compensated, and their testimony is often given intense media coverage. Given that context, expert testimony is often assumed to be crucial if not decisive in the outcomes of the cases in which it is offered. My 30-plus years of forensic work, which includes the cases described in this book, has led me to suspect that often the influence of expert witnesses (myself included) is not as great as many people seem to think.

As already noted, most of these cases and most others involving expert testimony feature dueling experts with competing opinions, each of which is generally plausible, especially to a lay jury. Thus, jurors must either decide which expert to believe or—as more often happens—find some other basis on which to reach a verdict. But beyond the battle of the experts, in many cases, including several detailed in this book, the alleged facts are so compelling (generally so compellingly awful) that no quantum of expert testimony, however well reasoned and presented, is likely to sway a jury. Consider the cases of Waneta Hoyt (who allegedly murdered five of her own children; Chapter 1), Charline Brundidge (who killed her abusive husband while he was making a tape-recorded phone call to 911; Chapter 2), Judith Neelley (who injected a 13-year-old with drain cleaner and then shot her to death when the caustic chemical failed to kill the child; Chapter 7), and Felicia Morgan (who killed a teenage peer allegedly in the course of a street robbery; Chapter 10). Although, in my estimation, my opinions in each of these cases were sound and amply supported by the evidence, I never expected that the triers of fact (jury or judge) would accept them and respond favorably to the defendants' claims.

A third lesson from the cases in this book, however, is that the testimony of forensic psychologists sometimes works in unanticipated ways. My testimony in Charline Brundidge's trial did not sway the jury but it did seem to have some impact on the judge, and it apparently influenced the governor, who later granted Charline clemency and cited my testimony. Similarly my testimony was part of the record that the governor of Alabama reviewed before deciding to commute Judy Neelley's death sentence. And I believe that my testimony on behalf of Felicia Morgan, though not sufficiently persuasive at trial, ultimately helped convince the trial judge to impose the most lenient sentence possible under the law.

A final lesson taught by these 10 cases relates to how lawyers regard and shape expert testimony. Most attorneys view expert testimony as a tool, a means to an end, a way of adding support to the cases they are trying to make on behalf of their clients. Attorneys are advocates, whereas experts (except for that small handful of hired guns briefly discussed earlier) are objective professionals who bring their expertise to bear in the search for truth and let the chips fall where they may. These differences in viewpoint between lawyers and experts have several important implications.

First, as has already been emphasized, forensic psychological experts retained by defense counsel often—in my case, usually—have no role in a case beyond conducting an evaluation and reporting the results to the attorney. Attorneys, as advocates, are—rightly so—more interested in vindicating their clients' rights than they are in getting at the truth of the matter.

Second, expert testimony is not a lecture but a carefully prepared dialogue controlled not by the expert but by the attorney, the court, and the rules of evidence. Thus, even when my testimony or that of any other expert witness is presented in court, it is shaped largely by the questions attorneys ask and the manner in which they ask those questions.

Direct examination is more predictable but still often frustrating for the expert witness because the attorney as advocate often wishes to limit the expert's testimony to that which is helpful while minimizing or omitting references to portions of the expert's views that do not support the client's defense.

Cross-examination on both sides, as was seen throughout this book, all too often is aimed at irrelevant issues, personal attacks on the expert, and a general effort to undermine the expert's credibility rather than to grapple directly and honestly with the expert's opinion and the bases for that opinion. The cross-examinations of me conducted by the prosecutors in the Brundidge, Justice (Chapter 4), and Manzella (Chapter 9) cases are perhaps the clearest examples of this common approach of attacking the messenger instead of the message.

Despite these and other limitations that have been amply illustrated in the cases described in this book, there can be little doubt that the expert testimony of forensic psychologists is generally regarded as a necessary and valuable tool in modern litigation, whether criminal or civil. Indeed, in many areas of the law, it is now difficult to imagine some kinds of trials without such testimony. As these cases also illustrate, however, and as anyone who has read this book with a critical eye can see, there is much room for improvement in the professional work of experts and attorneys who deal with forensic psychological issues. I hope that this modest volume and the lessons it conveys will contribute to an improvement in the quality of such work and its ultimate value to our system of justice.

Notes

Chapter 1: Waiver of *Miranda* Rights and Voluntary versus Coerced Confession

1. Alfred Steinschneider, "Prolonged Apnea and the Sudden Infant Death Syndrome: Clinical and Laboratory Observations," *Pediatrics* 50 (October 1972): 646–654.
2. J. F. Hick, "Sudden Infant Death Syndrome and Child Abuse," *Pediatrics* 52 (July 1973): 147–148.
3. Vincent J. M. DiMaio and Charles G. Bernstein, "A Case of Infanticide," *Journal of Forensic Sciences* 19 (October 1974): 744–754.
4. *Id.*
5. Dominick DiMaio and Vincent J. DiMaio, *Forensic Pathology* (Boca Raton, FL: CRC Press, 1993).
6. Richard Firstman and Jamie Talan, *The Death of Innocents* (New York: Bantam Books, 1997), 64.
7. Charles Hickey, Todd Lighty, and John O'Brien, *Goodbye My Little Ones* (New York: Penguin Books, 1996), 193.
8. Firstman and Talan, *supra* note 6, 116.

9. *Id.* at 138.
10. Hickey, Lighty, and O'Brien, *supra* note 7, 223.
11. *Id.*
12. Firstman and Talan, *supra* note 6, 146–147.
13. *Id.*
14. Statement signed by Waneta Hoyt on New York State police form dated March 23, 1994, p. 3.
15. Firstman and Talan, *supra* note 6, 434.
16. *Id.* at 547.
17. *Supra* note 14 at p. 1.
18. Transcript, statement of Waneta Hoyt, March 23, 1994, pp. 2–3.
19. American Psychiatric Association, *Diagnostic and Statistical Manual of Mental Disorders,* 4th ed. (Washington, DC: American Psychiatric Association, 1994), 665–666.
20. Firstman and Talan, *supra* note 6, 479.
21. *Id.*
22. Gisli Gudjonsson, personal communication, January 6, 1998.
23. Hickey, Lighty, and O'Brien, *supra* note 7, 325.
24. Trial transcript, quoted in Firstman and Talan, *supra* note 6, 558.
25. *Id.*
26. Trial transcript, quoted in Hickey, Lighty, and O'Brien, *supra* note 7, 344.
27. Hickey, Lighty, and O'Brien, *supra* note 7, 344.
28. Trial transcript, quoted in Hickey, Lighty, and O'Brien, *supra* note 7, 353.
29. Hickey, Lighty, and O'Brien, *supra* note 7, 373.
30. *Id.*
31. Firstman and Talan, *supra* note 6, 583.

Chapter 2: Battered Woman Syndrome, Self-Defense, and Extreme Emotional Disturbance

1. John O'Brien, "Juror lied, wife claims: Slayer of husband wants guilty verdict overturned," *Rochester Democrat and Chronicle,* November 22, 1986, 1B.

2. *Id.*
3. *Id.*
4. John O'Brien, "Husband Denies Lying as a Juror about Abuse: Convicted Woman Seeking New Trial," *Rochester Democrat and Chronicle,* December 19, 1986, 1B.
5. *Id.*
6. O'Brien, *supra,* note 1.
7. O'Brien, *supra,* note 4.
8. Rochelle D. Lewis, "Overturning of Murder Conviction Called 'rare,' " *Rochester Times-Union,* January 21, 1987.
9. *People v. Brundidge,* 526 N.Y.S.2d 407 (1988).
10. Charles Patrick Ewing, *Battered Women Who Kill* (Lexington MA: Lexington Books, 1987).
11. See, e.g., Lenore E. Walker, *The Battered Woman* (New York: Harper, 1980); Lenore E. Walker, *The Battered Woman Syndrome* (New York: Springer, 1984, 2000); Charles Patrick Ewing, *supra,* note 10; Angela Browne, *When Battered Women Kill* (New York: Simon & Schuster, 1989).
12. *State v. Kelly,* 478 A.2d 364, 377 (N.J. 1984).
13. Audiotape, 911 call from Marvin Brundidge, admitted into evidence in *People v. Brundidge,* indictment no. 803-85, Monroe County Court.
14. Trial transcript, *People v. Brundidge,* indictment no. 803-85, Monroe County Court, 704–719.
15. *Id.* at 747–759.
16. *Id.* at 768–777.
17. *Id.* at 778.
18. *Id.*
19. *Id.* at 965.
20. *Id.* at 878.
21. *Id.*
22. *Id.* at 1179–1180.
23. *Id.* at 1290–1292.
24. Winifred Yu, "Woman Who Killed Husband after a Beating Seeks Clemency," *Albany Times Union,* December 15, 1996, D1.

25. Jane Gross, "A New Life Opens, After Prison and Battering," *New York Times,* February 18, 1997, B1.

Chapter 3: Insanity: Malingering versus Organic Brain Syndrome

1. Kent Davy, "Doctor: Rouse Not Mentally Responsible," *Auburn Citizen,* January 13, 1989, 1, 3.
2. Trial transcript, *People v. Rouse,* State of New York, Cayuga County Court, indictment no. 3555 (January 9–13, 1989), 191.
3. *Id.*
4. *Id.* at 193.
5. *Id.* at 252.
6. *Id.* at 195.
7. *Id.*
8. *Id.* at 450.
9. *Id.* at 349.
10. *Id.* at 348–349.
11. *Id.* at 362–363.
12. *Id.* at 382–383, 387.
13. *Id.* at 400.
14. *Id.* at 401.
15. *Id.* at 402.
16. *Id.*
17. *Id.* at 416–417.
18. *Id.* at 422–425.
19. *Id.* at 456.
20. *Id.* at 457–458.
21. *Id.* at 459–460.
22. *Id.* at 465–466.
23. *Id.* at 486–487.
24. *Id.* at 497–498.
25. *Id.* at 522.
26. *Id.*
27. *Id.* at 523.
28. *Id.* at 382.

29. *Id.* at 541–542.
30. *Id.* at 542.
31. *Id.* at 544–549.
32. *Id.* at 551–552.
33. *Id.* at 550.
34. *Id.* at 555–556.
35. *Id.* at 569–570.
36. *Id.* at 571–574.
37. *Id.* at 579–580.
38. *Id.* at 608–612.
39. *Id.* at 623–624.
40. *Id.* at 645–647.
41. Nancy Ward, "Tillman's Murderer Gets the Maximum," *Auburn Citizen,* January 19, 1989, 1.

Chapter 4: Insanity, Extreme Emotional Disturbance, or Both?

1. Joshua Hammer, "Driven by His Long-Buried Rage, a 17-Year-Old Honor Student Lethally Lashes Out at His Family," *People,* November 18, 1985, 127.
2. Letter from Peter G. Pavlakis to Hon. Joseph Forma, December 11, 1986, appended to Presentence Memorandum, *People v. Justice,* indictment no. 85-1388-001, State of New York, Erie County Court.
3. Brief for Appellant, *People v. Justice,* indictment no. 85-1388-001, State of New York, Appellate Division, Fourth Department (October 19, 1993), 16.
4. Joshua Hammer, *supra* note 1.
5. Transcript, trial testimony of Charles Patrick Ewing, *People v. Justice,* indictment no. 85-1388-001, State of New York, Erie County Court (1992), 731.
6. *Id.*
7. *Id.*
8. *Id.* at 734.
9. Statement of John D. Justice, appended to Town of Tonawanda police department report, September 16, 1985, 1.

10. *Id.*
11. *Id.* at 2.
12. Transcript, trial testimony of Jin-Soo Rhee, MD, *People v. Justice,* indictment no. 85-1388-001, State of New York, Erie County Court (1986), 236.
13. Transcript, trial testimony of Emanuel Tanay, MD, *People v. Justice,* indictment no. 85-1388-001, State of New York, Erie County Court (1986), 648.
14. *Id.*
15. *Id.*
16. *Id.* at 686.
17. *Id.* at 740–741.
18. *Id.* at 750.
19. See *People v. Ivey,* 443 N.Y.S.2d 452, 453 (1981).
20. Transcript, trial testimony of Emanuel Tanay, *supra* note 13 at 798.
21. *Id.* at 808.
22. *Id.* at 856–857.
23. *Id.* at 857.
24. *Id.* at 824.
25. *Id.* at 898.
26. Transcript, trial testimony of Russell Barton, *People v. Justice,* indictment no. 85-1388-001, State of New York, Erie County Court (1986), 982.
27. *Id.* at 983.
28. *Id.*
29. *Id.* at 983–984.
30. *Id.* at 988.
31. *Id.* at 938–939.
32. *Id.* at 987.
33. *Id.*
34. *Id.* at 1005–1007.
35. *Id.* at 1010.
36. *Id.*
37. *Id.* at 1028.
38. *Id.* at 1062–1063.

39. American Psychiatric Association, *The Principles of Medical Ethics with Annotations Especially Applicable to Psychiatry* (Washington, DC: American Psychiatric Association, 2006), 4(13).
40. Transcript, trial testimony of Russell Barton, *supra* note 126 at 1063.
41. *Id.* at 1065.
42. *Id.* at 1066.
43. *Id.* at 1066–1067.
44. *Id.* at 1078.
45. *Id.* at 1078–1079.
46. *Id.* at 1079.
47. *Id.* at 1092.
48. *Id.* at 1080–1081.
49. *Id.* at 1160.
50. *Id.*
51. *Id.* at 1160–1171.
52. *People v. Justice,* 579 N.Y.S.2d 502, 504 (1991).
53. Tom Buckham, "Prosecutors Urge Ex-Kenmore Man to Plead Guilty in '85 Murders," *Buffalo News,* February 4, 1992, B1.
54. *Id.*
55. Transcript, trial testimony of Charles Patrick Ewing, *People v. Justice,* indictment no. 85-1388-001, State of New York, Erie County Court (1992), 796–798.
56. *Id.* at 1297–1298.
57. *Id.* at 1310–1312.
58. *Id.* at 1312.
59. *Id.* at 1322–1323.
60. *Id.* at 1324–1326.
61. *Id.* at 1420–1421.

Chapter 5: Voluntary or Coerced Confession?

1. Rebecca Coffer, *God Cop, Bad Cop: A True Story of Murder and Mayhem* (Far Hills, NJ: New Horizon Press, 1994), 124.
2. *Id.* at 160.

3. *Id.*
4. Transcript, statement of Shirley Kinge to New York State police, February 7, 1990, 2.
5. *Id.* at 3.
6. *Id.*
7. *Id.* at 4; See also Deborah Homsher, *From Blood to Verdict* (Ithaca, NY: McBooks, 1993), 78.
8. *Id.* at 78–79.
9. Coffer, *supra* note 1 at 188.
10. Affirmation of William P. Sullivan, Jr., *People v. Kinge,* indictment no. 90-022 (Tompkins County Court, undated).
11. Coffer, *supra* note 1 at 166.
12. *Id.* at 167.
13. *Id.* at 170.
14. Transcript, pretrial testimony of H. Karl Chandler, *People v. Kinge,* indictment no. 90-022 (Tompkins County Court, 1992), 228.
15. *Id.* at 228, 338.
16. Coffer, *supra* note 1 at 175.
17. *Id.* at 202.
18. *Id.* at 205.
19. Thomas Fine, "Jury Can't Hear of Kinge's Mental State," *Syracuse Post-Standard,* November 6, 1990, B1.
20. *In the Matter of Sullivan,* 586 N.Y.S.2d 322, 323 (1992).
21. Coffer, *supra* note 1 at 208.
22. *Id.*
23. *Id.* at 207.
24. *Id.* at 211.
25. *Id.*
26. *In the Matter of Sullivan, supra* note 20 at 326.
27. Coffer, *supra* note 1 at 230.
28. *Id.* at 238.
29. *Id.* at 242.
30. *Id.* at 261.
31. Thomas Fine, "Trooper Sentenced to 2–6 Years," *Syracuse Post-Standard,* December 17, 1992, A1.
32. *Id.*

33. Thomas Fine, "Harding Apologizes at Ithaca Sentencing but the Ex-Trooper, Who Will Spend up to 12 Years in Prison for Faking Evidence, Says He Thought His Victims 'Were Dangerous,'" *Syracuse Post-Standard,* December 17, 1992, A1.

34. *Id.*

35. Rebecca James, "Harding Admits Fakery in 5th Case: As the Former Investigator Is Sentenced to Prison, He Says Others Share the Blame," *Syracuse Post-Standard,* January 6, 1993, A1.

Chapter 6: Child Abuse Victim, Sexual Predator, or Both?

1. Trial transcript of Charles Patrick Ewing, *People v. William Shrubsall,* indictment no. 88-148, Niagara County Court, August 29, 1988, 74.

2. Transcript, statement of William Shrubsall to Niagara Falls police, 36–41.

3. *Id.* at 42–43.

4. Charles Patrick Ewing, *Battered Women Who Kill* (Lexington MA: Lexington Books, 1987), 79.

5. David Margolick, "Law Professor to Administer Courts in State," *New York Times,* February 1, 1985, B2.

6. Louise Continelli, "Why Kids Kill," *Buffalo News Magazine,* April 1, 1990, 6, 9–13.

7. *Id.* at 12.

8. *People v. Shrubsall,* 562 N.Y.S.2d 290 (1990), 292.

9. "Shrubsall a Stellar Parolee after Release from Prison, Halifax Hearing Told," *Canadian Press Newswire,* March 27, 2001.

10. Dan Herbeck and Gene Warner, "Did the System Fail? Bitter Debate Sparked by the Violent Aftermath of Shrubsall's Release after 16 Months in Prison," *Buffalo News,* August 3, 1998, 1A.

11. Paul Westmoore, "Despite Suicide Note, Shrubsall Still Sought as Fugitive in Sex Attack," *Buffalo News,* April 24, 1998, 1B.

12. Steven Watson and Gene Warner, "The Secret Life of a Predator during Two Years on the Run," *Buffalo News,* August 2, 1998, 1A.

13. *Id.*

14. *Regina v. Shrubsall,* 2002 W.C.B.J 13524, 101 (Nova Scotia Supreme Court, 2001).
15. "Shrubsall Had Look of Hatred for Women after Alleged Attack: Witness," *Canadian Press Newswire,* March 21, 2001.
16. *Id.*
17. "Shrubsall Lost Control after Too Much Mothering, Halifax Court Told," *Canadian Press Newswire,* October 1, 2001.
18. *Id.*
19. "Shrubsall Attacked Boy Who Beat His Video Game Score, Halifax Court Told," *Canadian Press Newswire,* March 8, 2001.
20. "Women Describe Attacks by Convicted Murderer," *Toronto Star,* March 20, 2001, 1.
21. "Shrubsall a Psychopath Who Will Offend All His Life, Halifax Court Told," *Canadian Press Newswire,* March 20, 2001.
22. *Id.*
23. *Id.*
24. *People v. Shrubsall,* 562 N.Y.S.2d 290, 292 (1990).
25. American Psychiatric Association, *Diagnostic and Statistical Manual of Mental Disorders,* 4th ed. (Washington, DC: American Psychiatric Association, 1994), 645.
26. *Regina v. Shrubsall,* 2002 W.C.B.J. 13524, 203 (Nova Scotia Supreme Court, 2001).
27. *Id.* at 209.
28. *Id.* at 229–233.
29. Dan Herbeck and Gene Warner, *supra* note 10.

Chapter 7: Battered Woman Syndrome, Duress, and the Death Penalty

1. Transcript, trial testimony of Jo Ann Browning, *State v. Neelley,* DeKalb County Circuit Court, case no. CC-82-276 (1983), cited in Appellant's Brief in Support of Petition for Writ of Certiorari to the court of Criminal Appeals of the State of Alabama, *State v. Neelley,* 107.
2. Trial testimony, Jo Ann Browning, *State v. Neelley,* DeKalb County Circuit Court, case no. CC-82-276 (1983), cited in Thomas H.

Cook, *Early Graves* (New York: Dutton/Penguin Books, 1990), 232–233.

3. Contrasting photographs are available in Cook, *supra* note 2 between p. 146 and p. 147.

4. Trial testimony of Judith Ann Neelley, *State v. Neelley,* DeKalb County Circuit Court, case no. CC-82-276 (1983), cited in Thomas H. Cook, *Early Graves* (New York: Dutton/Penguin Books, 1990), 254.

5. *Id*. at 255.

6. *Id*. at 260.

7. *Id*. at 268.

8. *Id*. at 269.

9. *Id*. at 269–270.

10. Trial testimony of Alexander A. Salillas, MD, *State v. Neelley,* DeKalb County Circuit Court, case no. CC-82-276 (1983), cited in Appellant's Brief in Support of Petition for Writ of Certiorari to the court of Criminal Appeals of the State of Alabama, *State v. Neelley,* 204.

11. *Id*. at 208.

12. Trial testimony of Alexander A. Salillas, MD, *State v. Neelley,* DeKalb County Circuit Court, case no. CC-82-276 (1983), cited in Thomas H. Cook, *Early Graves* (New York: Dutton/Penguin Books, 1990), 275.

13. *Id*. at 276.

14. Closing argument of Robert French Esq., *State v. Neelley,* DeKalb County Circuit Court, case no. CC-82-276 (1983), cited in Thomas H. Cook, *Early Graves* (New York: Dutton/Penguin Books, 1990), 290.

15. Sentencing Remarks of Hon. Randal Cole, *State v. Neelley,* DeKalb County Circuit Court, case no. CC-82-276 (1983), cited in Thomas H. Cook, *Early Graves* (New York: Dutton/Penguin Books, 1990), 293–294.

16. Darell Norman, "Expert says Mrs. Neeley 'was a robot,' " *Fort Payne Times-Journal,* August 15–16, 1987, 1.

17. *Id.*

18. *Id.*

19. Tom Gordon, "Neelley's Actions Triggered by Abuse, Psychologist Testifies," *Birmingham News,* August 15, 1987, A3.
20. Decision of Hon. Randall Cole, *People v. Neelley,* DeKalb County Circuit Court, case no. CC-82-276 (1987).
21. *Ex parte Judith Ann Neelley,* 642 So. 2d 510 (1994).
22. Scott Wright, "Fob James Discusses Neelley Sentence Commutation," *Post* (Cherokee County, AL), July 22, 2002, 1.
23. *Id.*
24. "Ex-Husband Says Neelley Still Dangerous," *Birmingham News,* February 22, 1999, 3B.
25. *Id.*

Chapter 8: Validation of Alleged Child Sexual Abuse

1. *People v. Duell,* 558 N.Y.S.2d 395, 396 (1990).
2. Transcript, trial testimony of Becky Wendt, *People v. Knupp,* indictment no. 89-1-013, Ontario County Court (1989), 36–39.
3. Transcript, pretrial testimony of Becky Wendt, *People v. Knupp,* indictment no. 89-1-013, Ontario County Court (1989), 20.
4. *Id.*
5. *Id.* at 28.
6. Transcript, trial testimony of Katherine Knupp, *People v. Knupp,* indictment no. 89-1-013, Ontario County Court (1989), 123.
7. *Id.* at 128.
8. *Id.* at 131.
9. *Id.* at 132.
10. *Id.* at 133.
11. *Id.* at 134.
12. *Id.* at 149.
13. *Id.* at 128.
14. *Id.* at 129.
15. *Id.*
16. *Id.* at 135.
17. Transcript, trial testimony of Faith Knupp, *People v. Knupp,* indictment no. 89-1-013, Ontario County Court (1989), 170–171.

18. Transcript, trial testimony of Becky Wendt, *People v. Knupp,* indictment no. 89-1-013, Ontario County Court (1989), 42–45.

19. *Id.* at 48.

20. *Id.*

21. *Id.* at 53.

22. *Id.* at 60.

23. *Id.* at 61–63.

24. *Id.* at 64.

25. *Id.* at 69.

26. *Id.*

27. *Id.* at 69–70.

28. *Id.* at 71.

29. *Id.*

30. Jack Jones, "Dad Jailed as 'Sex Animal' but Serious Doubts Linger," *Rochester Democrat and Chronicle,* August 27, 1989, 1A, 6A.

31. *Id.*

32. *Id.*

33. *Id.*

34. *Id.*

35. *Id.*

36. *Id.*

37. "A Miscarriage of Justice," *Rochester Democrat and Chronicle,* December 19, 1989, 12A.

38. *People v. Duell,* 558 N.Y.S.2d 395, 396 (1990).

39. *People v. Knupp,* 579 N.Y.S.2d 801, 802–803 (1992).

40. Jack Jones, "Knupp Denies Sexually Abusing Kids," *Rochester Democrat and Chronicle,* April 21, 1992, 1A, 4A.

41. *Id.*

42. Joel Freedman, "Richard Knupp Acquitted," *Justicia: Newsletter of Greater Rochester Community of Churches Judicial Process Commission,* June 1992, 1.

43. Transcript, trial testimony of Charles Patrick Ewing, *People v. Knupp,* indictment no. 89-1-013, Ontario County Court (1992), 11.

44. *Id.* at 11–12.

45. *Id.* at 20–21.
46. *Id.* at 13.
47. *Id.* at 16.
48. *Id.*
49. *Id.* at 16–17.
50. *Id.* at 17.
51. *Id.*
52. *Id.* at 39.

Chapter 9: Murder or Manslaughter? Extreme Emotional Disturbance

1. Transcript, trial testimony of Charles Patrick Ewing, *People v. Manzella,* indictment no. 89-1747, New York State Supreme Court, Erie County (1991), 47.
2. *Id.* at 48.
3. *Id.*
4. *Id.*
5. *Id.*
6. *Id.*
7. *Id.*
8. *Id.*
9. *Id.* at 49.
10. *Id.* at 61.
11. *Id.* at 48.
12. *Id.* at 64–65.
13. *Id.* at 65.
14. Transcript, taped conversation between Rudolph Manzella and Officers Dennis Rankin and Robert Woods, October 20, 1989 (Vol. C-1), 3–5.
15. Transcript, trial testimony of Ewing, *supra* note 1 at 18–20.
16. *Id.* at 21.
17. Alan S. Kaufman, 2003, *Practice Effects,* www.speechandlanguage.com/cafe/13.asp. (accessed January 29, 2008).
18. Transcript, trial testimony Ewing, *supra* note 1 at 31.
19. *Id.* at 33–34.

20. *Id.* at 36–37.
21. *Id.* at 37.
22. *Id.* at 50.
23. *Id.* at 54.
24. *Id.* at 58.
25. *Id.* at 1051–1052.
26. *Id.* at 322.
27. *Id.* at 333.
28. *Id.* at 334.
29. *Id.*
30. *Id.* at 335–336.
31. *Id.* at 338.
32. *Id.* at 339.
33. *Id.* at 340–341.
34. *Id.* at 348–349.
35. Testimony, Russell Barton, cited in Brief and Appendix for Appellant, *People v. Manzella,* indictment no. 88-1747 (State of New York, Appellate Division, Fourth Department, March 11, 1993), 14.
36. *Id.* at 15.
37. *Id.* at 33.
38. *Id.* at 33–34.
39. *Id.* at 34.

Chapter 10: Insanity, Posttraumatic Stress Disorder, and Brief Reactive Psychosis

1. Charles Patrick Ewing, *Kids Who Kill* (Lexington MA: Lexington Books, 1990); Charles Patrick Ewing, *When Children Kill: The Dynamics of Juvenile Homicide* (Lexington MA: Lexington Books, 1990).
2. Transcript, trial testimony of Charles Patrick Ewing, *State v. Morgan,* case no. F-920915, State of Wisconsin, Milwaukee County Circuit Court (1992), 1775.
3. *Id.*
4. *Id.*

5. "An Excuse to Kill," *ABC NEWS 20/20,* May 27, 1994 (transcript no. 1421).
6. *State v. Morgan,* 536 N.W.2d 425, 428 (1995).
7. *Id.*
8. *Id.*
9. *Id.*
10. *Id.* at 429.
11. American Psychiatric Association, *Diagnostic and Statistical Manual of Mental Disorders,* 3rd ed., rev. (Washington, DC: American Psychiatric Association, 1987), 205.
12. *Id.* at 206.
13. Elissa P. Benedek and Dewey G. Cornell (Eds.), *Juvenile Homicide* (Washington, DC: American Psychiatric Publishing, 1989).
14. American Psychiatric Association, *supra* note 11 at 346.
15. *Morgan v. Krenke,* 72 F. Supp. 2d 980, 988 (1999).
16. *Id.* at 990.
17. *Id.* at 991.
18. *Id.* at 1019–1020.
19. Transcript, trial testimony of Charles Patrick Ewing, *supra* note 2 at 1763–1765.
20. *Id.* at 1765–1766.
21. *Id.* at 1767.
22. *Id.* at 1804–1805.
23. *Morgan v. Krenke,* 72 F. Supp. 2d 980, 1019 (1999).
24. *State v. Morgan,* 536 N.W.2d 425, 446 (1995).
25. "An Excuse to Kill," *supra* note 5.
26. *Id.*
27. *Id.*
28. *State v. Morgan,* 536 N.W.2d 425, 439 (1995).
29. *Id.* at 453.
30. *Id.* at 451.
31. *Id.* at 436.
32. *Id.* at 449.
33. *Morgan v. Krenke,* 72 F. Supp. 2d 980, 1008–1014 (1999).
34. *Morgan v. Krenke,* 232 F.3d 562, 568–569 (2000).

INDEX

C

D

E

F

G

H

J

K

L

M

N

P

Q

R